SAVING ABIGAIL GRACE

SAVING ABIGAIL GRACE

A Mother's Story of Transforming Pain into Purpose

LAYLA SLATER

www.SavingAbigailGrace.com

First edition

ISBN: 979-8-9912357-0-9 (Paperback)
ISBN: 979-8-9912357-1-6 (Hardcover)
ISBN: 979-8-9912357-2-3 (eBook)

Library of Congress Control Number: 2024915688

Book coach: Bonnie B. Daneker
www.TheAuthorsGreenhouse.com

Editor: Ivette Maymi
www.PolishedPagesEditorial.com

Cover Design and Interior Formatting: Becky's Graphic Design,® LLC
www.BeckysGraphicDesign.com

Printed in the United States of America

To my dad, Gerard P. Paulus

This book is dedicated to the memory of the man who held my hand through childhood, cheered me on through my toughest teen moments, and beamed with pride over the woman I became. Never allowing me to give in to my fears or self-doubts, he taught me to be tougher than I believed with his unwavering faith in me and my abilities. My dad and mom raised a timid little girl into a woman who chases dreams because they taught me that anything was within reach with hard work and determination.

Dad, I love you more than ever, miss you every day, and look forward to the day when I can see you again for eternity.

You always have been and forever will be my Superman!

Foreword

I was honored when Layla asked me to contribute to this publication about their family's experiences and lessons learned throughout Abi's difficult medical and educational journey. Layla's book will be an inspiring and valuable resource for all parents whose children encounter medical and educational challenges.

When I first met the Slater family, I had been a school psychologist since 1977 with experiences including consultation and diagnostic responsibilities in public and parochial schools and in a research project studying the cognitive development of children who had been in the Neonatal Intensive Care Unit in a local children's hospital. The combination of these experiences led to my appreciation of the plasticity and adaptability of a young child's brain and the value of early interventions. My involvement with Abi's education definitely solidified this conviction.

I vividly remember the day Layla and Brian walked into the conference room for their first of many meetings with our special education team at Abi's elementary school. They bravely but anxiously smiled, graciously greeted all the members of our group, sat down at the table, and we began the discussion and the process that would provide Abi with the support and the resources she would need.

My impressions from that first meeting were confirmed throughout the many years we worked together. First, Layla and Brian were always very well prepared and knowledgeable about Abi's fluctuating and sometimes terrifying medical challenges.

They were realistic but also optimistic about Abi's possible outcomes. Second, as important members of the team, Layla and Brian understood the value of a cooperative working relationship with the school staff. Their well-informed contributions and opinions provided our team with direction and support. Finally, while Abi's amazing success has been the result of her own perseverance, confidence, and positivity, these traits were modeled and encouraged by her parents. There is no substitute for the love, faith, devotion, and advocacy of parents.

Saving Abigail Grace will take the reader on a roller coaster ride of Abi's early years and will provide insight, valuable resources, and hope for all. Spoiler alert: there is a happy ending!

—Karen Zichterman
Retired School Psychologist for District 321 and member
of Abigail's Special Education Team

Contents

Foreword vii

Introduction 1

CHAPTER 1   Two Semis, One Helicopter, and a Shattered Plan 3

CHAPTER 2   Spanish Class, Donuts, and Pursuit of the White Picket Fence 13

CHAPTER 3   The ICU Giant and Her Invalid Mother 31

CHAPTER 4   The Carolyn Scott Rainbow House 51

CHAPTER 5   Back Home. . . Or So We Thought 71

CHAPTER 6   A New "Normal" 87

CHAPTER 7   Hometown Humble Pie 95

CHAPTER 8   Doctors, Specialists, and Therapists, Oh My! 107

CHAPTER 9   Faith and Firsts 117

CHAPTER 10   PT, OT, CTs, EEGs, and IEPs: What the Heck Are These? 143

CHAPTER 11   School Daze 165

CHAPTER 12   Seizures, Celebrations, and Saying Goodbye 177

CHAPTER 13   Growing Forward and Healing Together 213

Acknowledgments 245

About the Author 247

Glossary 249

Introduction

LIFE IS A WILD RIDE, full of twists and turns we never see coming. But there is one thing we can count on: sooner or later, we all experience some sort of trauma. How we choose to react to that trauma is what makes us who we are. Will we shatter like glass, or become a diamond under the pressure?

What you're about to dive into is my story of transforming my darkest day into a beacon of hope. This isn't just about reliving the horrors of October 17, 2002 — it's about rising from the ashes through determination and resilience. If you're reading this, chances are my journey will somehow resonate with you, even if our paths have not unfolded in the same way.

Maybe you've faced the screech of tires and the crunch of metal, the beep of NICU hospital machines, or the warm embrace of a hospitality house. Perhaps you've advocated for your child in Individualized Education Program (IEP) meetings, or held their hand through the terror of seizures, surgeries, diagnoses, or the challenges of a body that works differently. Maybe your faith is eluding you, you're lacking inspiration, or you long to feel like you are not alone.

I hope these pages offer you more than just words. My desire is that they will give you the strength to keep going, the comfort of knowing you're not alone, and the spark of faith when it flickers. Because I mostly stumbled every step of the way through my experience, the resources that I have offered in this book are my way of saving you at least some of the same struggles.

Inside each chapter, you will find a chronology of my

experience over the past two decades, accompanied by my advice and resources to assist you in learning more about becoming the advocate that your child needs. These "sidebars," as I have called them, include resources that I wish I would have had on my pre-technology trip through the most difficult years of my life.

Whatever brought you to my story, I pray that the precious time you have spent with these pages in your hands has been time well spent — that my words make you stronger, inspire you to keep rising, and remind you that even in the darkest times, there is always hope. There will be stormy days, so I encourage you to never give up and to always keep the end goal in the front seat while you clutch the steering wheel with white knuckles, because one day, those dark clouds will only be visible from your rearview mirror.

Thank you for trusting me on your personal journey.

—Layla

CHAPTER ONE

Two Semis, One Helicopter, and a Shattered Plan

STUNNED BY THE IMPACT AND overwhelming stench of rubber, I came back to consciousness as the paramedic swiftly pushed away the chalky, inflated airbag that blew up in my face moments before.

"How far along are you?"

A woman's voice, calm but authoritative, came from the driver's side of my 2001 silver Pontiac Grand Am. Pinned by the pieces of the passenger-side interior that had been crushed into the driver's seat, I could allow only my eyes to search for the source of the voice. When I finally locked eyes with her, the trepidation on her face told me it was far more dire than I could even imagine.

"You are obviously pregnant," she calmly observed. "Do you know how far along you are?" My interrogator, her voice almost angelic, seemed out of place from the chaotic scene that was unfolding around us.

Pregnant? I was so dazed that I had momentarily *forgotten* about the pregnancy. I stared down at my protruding midsection in horror, my mind reeling. Underneath me on the seat of my mangled new car, a pool of my blood was rapidly spreading. *What. . . how. . . oh my God!*

Extreme panic set in.

"Uh, I . . . I don't know!" I stammered, fear clawing at my throat.

"Where does it hurt?" she asked, her tone becoming more forceful with each word.

The anguished cries that escaped my battered body served as primal language the gathering crowd could understand. My consciousness grew hazy, my attempts at speech devolving into incoherent fragments. My voice was like a stranger's as I made every effort to form words.

The scene was chaotic: The otherwise clear, cool autumn sky was filled with black billowing smoke, and the asphalt of Highway 77, a two-lane rural highway outside of a small farming community called Wahoo, Nebraska, was littered with crash debris. The air pulsed with the frantic shouts of police, fire crews, and medics, their words tumbling out in desperate attempts to recount the heart-stopping moments that had just unfolded.

As the darkness closed in and I felt my life slipping away, so many thoughts were echoing through my mind like a scream: *What happened? Where is Noah? Is he dead? Am I going to die? What about the baby? I need my husband!*

This was not part of my perfect plan.

An Uneventful Start to the Day

I remember that Thursday morning well—October 17, 2002. It was like any other day that preceded it. My husband, Brian, and I woke up long before the sun would make its appearance to get ourselves and our son, Noah, ready for the workday. Like most American families, weekday mornings in the Slater home were typically busy and hurried. I had my routine dialed in and I did much of my preparation the prior evening (which meant our evenings were busy as well). The smell of freshly brewed coffee always filled the air of the main floor of our narrow three-story duplex, where a small kitchen, dining area, and living room were located. Each morning, I clumsily descended the two flights of stairs from my bedroom to the basement, where I knocked out my daily workout before waking my sandy-haired, blue-eyed toddler, Noah.

Because Brian liked to get a head start on the day before his employees arrived at work, he aimed to leave home by 6:00 most mornings, leaving me to prepare myself and Noah for the long day ahead of us. After Brian left, I climbed into a hot, steamy shower, and embraced the floral fragrance of my favorite body-wash while I contemplated the eight hours of work that lay ahead of me. My coworker, Marla, and I were to be out of the office working in a crop field, as we normally did, and the weather was to be decent for an autumn day in the Midwest. We worked as a team to take elevations of corn, bean, and wheat fields to design soil erosion practices such as terraces and basins. I loved that part of my job as a Soil Conservation Technician with the USDA Natural Resources Conservation Service (NRCS)—working with Marla outside instead of sitting behind cubicle walls.

Freshly energized from my shower, I quickly put on my maternity jeans and oversized sweatshirt, packed up our things, and headed out the door, right on time. I strapped Noah into his car seat, located in the backseat on the passenger side, and out of town we headed as the sun finally made its appearance. Our 40-minute commute from Lincoln to rural Wahoo allowed me time to men-

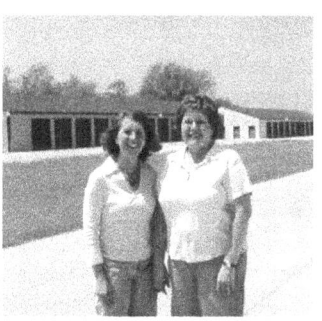

Me with Marla

tally prepare for the day and afforded us extra time to bond, so I enjoyed our drive together. When we reached Wahoo, I dropped Noah off at daycare, like I had many times before. The field office where I worked was only a short five-minute drive from there.

My Nightmare Begins

As usual, I drove toward the building where I had worked for only a few short months. I saw a red semitruck hauling a flatbed trailer approaching from the opposite direction, and I waited with my left turn signal blinking to indicate my intentions of entering the parking lot. That was the moment that separated my life as I knew it from what it was to become. Without noticing the commotion that had taken place directly behind my vehicle, I was violently thrust into the path of the red ravager after being hit from behind by another semitruck. Its driver would unwittingly be the terminator of my perfect paradigm—the creator of my hell on earth.

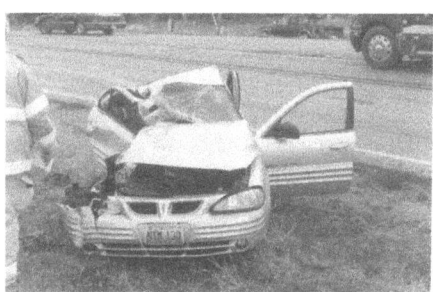
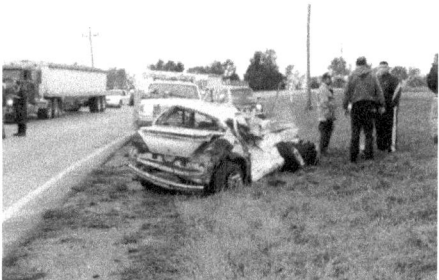
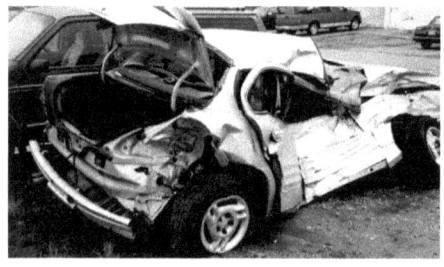
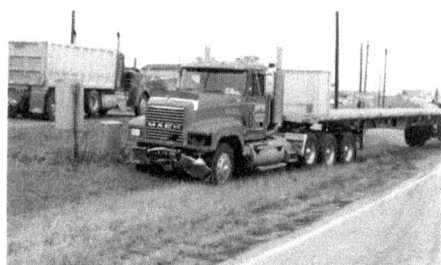
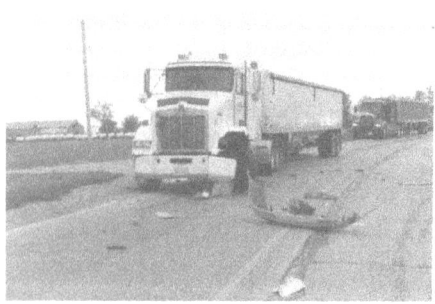
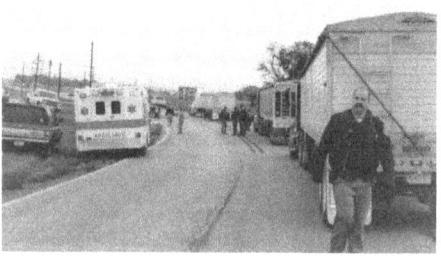

A cacophony of noises—a loud, jolting crash, shattering glass, squealing brakes, metal on metal, and my own moans and groans—were all I remember hearing for what seemed like an eternity but a flash at the same time. I clung to the steering wheel like my life depended upon it (in fact, it did). As my car careened and spun like a pinball in a life-sized arcade, I caught glimpses of various scenes flashing by—trees, my office building, other vehicles, and clouds scattered in the blue sky. It was like a chaotic movie playing out before my eyes until my car finally came to a stop several hundred feet away from where I was first struck.

Initially, confusion washed over me as I tried to process the fact that I had just been involved in a four-vehicle crash that would change my life forever. The next wave of emotions hit me like a ton of bricks: excruciating pain and unbearable discomfort, especially in my right hip.

The accident reconstruction report showed that while I was waiting for that big red monster to pass, the driver of a white pickup truck that was immediately behind me noticed in his rearview mirror a fast-approaching semitruck. And since my attention was in front of me, I hadn't a clue what was unfolding behind me. Naturally, the driver of the pickup swerved out of the way to avoid being sandwiched between my car and the white big rig behind him, leaving me to absorb most of the impact—lucky me. My car was violently struck from behind and since my steering wheel was already positioned to steer my car to the left, I was thrust into the path of the oncoming red semi that I would see in my nightmares for months to come.

Where is Noah?

Still disoriented, I realized that I was sitting in the only area of the vehicle that could accommodate a survivor, which threw me into a dazed state of alarm. My car had been mangled nearly beyond recognition, with all passenger seating compounded like an accordion.

"Where is my son?" I shrieked in terror, momentarily forgetting that I had dropped him off at daycare only moments before. "Tell me where my son is!" Fear coursed through me as I imagined the worst: my precious two-and-a-half-year-old son, dead in a roadside ditch with only pieces of his car seat left behind. The news that he wasn't in the car when I was hit didn't register with me; I was convinced they were just trying to keep me calm. My mind raced with thoughts of my son, unable to shake the fear that something terrible had happened to him.

My Incredible Coworkers

My coworkers were some of the first to arrive, followed by emergency personnel, who all had their own specific job to do. Some were there to make sure I did not lose consciousness, some to collect information from all parties involved, and some who witnessed the boisterous turning point of my tranquil life. There were some whose job was to rescue me from the wreckage and deliver me to the nearby hospital, and then there was the one poor police officer whose unfortunate job was to notify my husband of the episode.

While I had become preoccupied with the possibilities of what had happened to Noah, some of the men I knew from work were looking in the ditches and everywhere else in hopes not to find him.

I vaguely remember Marla and Jami, two coworkers, watching the determined emergency rescue team work feverishly to extract me from the ruins of my demolished Grand Am. The team carefully, but quickly, placed me on a stretcher before loading me into an ambulance. I was then whisked off to the local hospital where my coworkers were able to see firsthand the actuality of it all.

While I was being expedited to the Saunders County Community Hospital, Brian was already en route, contacted by the officer on the scene, and had a 40-minute drive (or an eternity, as he remembers it) to contemplate all the possibilities of what could have happened. Although I am grateful that he was notified, the gentleman who made that inevitable phone call left my stricken husband in limbo about what sort of scene he would be walking into. He was only told that his wife had been in a terrible accident and that he should come to the hospital right away. Of course, he was so shaken when he hung up the telephone at work that his coworkers deemed him unable to drive. One of them transported him frantically to the hospital to be with me. For all he knew, he would be greeted by the dead bodies of his wife, young son, and unborn child.

At the hospital, I remember being wheeled down a long, sterile corridor, much like what you would see in a movie. The clattering of the steel wheels of the stretcher, and the looks on my coworkers' faces while they hovered over me, will forever be a haunting memory. They all appeared emotionless, staring at me as if I were already a body in the morgue. Memory tells me that none of them had much of a response to my cries and screams, I am sure because they were in total shock at the sight of my banged-up body and the awful noises that were leaving it. I still have visions of my coworker Carol just standing there, grasping her purse while all the others stood with their arms folded. It was eerie.

StarCare Life Flight

With my head and neck immobilized, all I could see was the ceiling above me. As I was wheeled to an examination room down a hallway that seemed never ending, white lights continued to pass me overhead, one after another. I had always heard that when a person is on her way out of this world and into the afterlife, bright white lights appear. So I thought, *This is it; I am on my way to meet my maker.* I was utterly paralyzed with fear and anticipation, accompanied by intense pain like I had never felt before, primarily in my right hip and lower back.

Medical professionals were able to examine my mutilated body, and an ordered obstetric ultrasound shed light on the condition of the baby that was still active inside me. The team administered morphine since my pain was registering a 10 on a scale of 1 to 10. They also noticed that there was still massive drainage coming from my vaginal area, which indicated that something was seriously wrong with the pregnancy. While there were still fetal movements showing on a monitor, the team at Saunders County Community Hospital knew this case was one that they were not equipped to handle. After Brian and his coworker reached the hospital, the medical team decided that I, along with my baby in utero would be transferred via helicopter to Bryan Lincoln General Hospital (Bryan LGH).

Even after receiving the highest dose of morphine possible, the pain I experienced was unbearable. I was loaded into the StarCare helicopter like precious cargo, and we hurried on our way to the next destination. One of the only memories I have of this flight is of the gentle brunette nurse that accompanied me. "Looks like you're going to have a baby today," she said. "No, I'm not ready!" I shrieked. I worried at that point that if I delivered the baby that day, there would be only a small chance that he or she could survive. Being only 32 weeks into my pregnancy, this baby needed to grow for eight more weeks to be at full term. I was terrified!

While I, my unborn child, and our emergency medical team were in flight, a new team of specialists were rapidly assembling on the ground to ensure a smooth, delicate transition to our second hospital. After what seemed like an endless flight, the chopper landed atop Bryan LGH, where there was a team of trauma specialists eagerly awaiting my arrival. By this time, the morphine had dissipated, and the pain was again intolerable. As I remember, nearly every part of my body was in pain, but it was especially excruciating on my right side, the side that was hit when I was T-boned by the red semi. I complained to the team that I had insufferable pain in my neck, chest, right shoulder, right wrist, back, and right hip. My vaginal area was still bleeding and showing a heavy discharge, and the team decided that the baby was a priority. Since the fetal heart rate was still strong enough, they decided that it would be best to diagnose my injuries by using X-rays and CT scans.

My Diagnosis

What the doctors found explained why I felt such agonizing pain. Their technical reports read:

> "...*right-side sacral and left-side pubic fractures, multiple contusions around the buttocks and the right thigh, a right rotator cuff injury, a ligament tear in her right wrist, retroperitoneal hematoma, increasing pleural effusion, a very large hematoma of the left breast, chemosis, and a subchorionic placental hemorrhage.*"

In layperson's terms, I had suffered two pelvic fractures; multiple bruises, particularly in my backside and right thigh; injuries to my right shoulder and wrist; bleeding in the abdominal and pelvic cavities; fluid in the lungs; pooling blood and massive swelling on my left breast; swelling in my right eye; and internal bleeding that endangered my pregnancy. The continued bleeding was what troubled everyone the most; my placenta had detached from the wall of my uterus, and I was losing fluid that was vital to the baby's survival.

The painful result was that a fetal heart monitor revealed the baby's heart rate was weakening and steadily declining. The baby had to be delivered immediately via emergency cesarean section—there was no other option.

Due to the condition that I was in physically, I had no knowledge of the treacherous terrain that my unborn child had encountered. Also unbeknownst to me, everyone involved already knew that it was more than stress and harm that was coming her way. The baby that I was about to deliver was coming in a matter of minutes, totally unprepared for what he or she would have to endure for the rest of his or her life. Even worse, Brian and I were no more prepared than the baby was. Terrified and with consciousness failing me, I realized I had been given a passport to pain that would take my sweet new baby and me on a slow journey through hell.

To learn more about the medical terms and
topics discussed in this chapter, visit this link:

www.SavingAbigailGrace.com

CHAPTER TWO

Spanish Class, Donuts, and Pursuit of the White Picket Fence

BRIAN AND I MET IN Spanish class while attending Western Illinois University in 1995 and became well acquainted during the three-and-a-half-year friendship that we developed while there. Since Brian never had a vehicle, I gave him rides home after class or to Spanish labs, where we worked on our second language as partners. Hoping to become a police officer like his father, he majored in criminal justice, while I majored in geology with a love for environmental and earth sciences.

Brian was my buddy who always brought humor into every conversation we had, even when the subject matter was otherwise heavy. Speaking very little about his family or his feelings at first, Brian was a mystery, but I was intrigued by him. He stood 6'3" (compared to my 5'3"), had a football player's build with reddish-blond hair, and his smile revealed a small gap between his two front teeth. As big as he was and as intimidating as he could seem, I found his general disposition incredibly gentle. Unlike me, he was not at all concerned with pleasing others. I could tell when we were first getting to know each other that he was somewhat wounded, but it would take a long time to learn why.

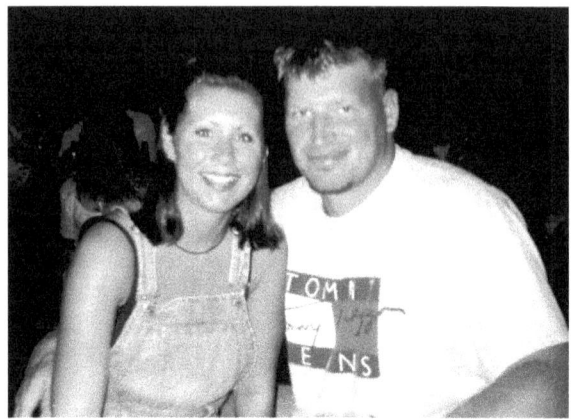

We had very different childhoods: mine was loving and nurturing, with both parents at home, while Brian's lacked parental support and guidance, having to learn at a very young age to be independent. His older sister, Tammy, was instrumental in his upbringing. As the oldest of the four children with an absent mother, she was responsible for her siblings' welfare for much of their childhood. As a result of his unstable childhood and feelings of abandonment, I initially found it difficult to break through the walls that he had built for protection.

Busy with my sorority and my own circle of friends, there never seemed to be a chance for Brian and me to become romantic, and although I suspected he might be interested in that type of relationship with me, I never wanted to jeopardize our friendship. My life was full of deadlines, executive board and chapter meetings, fraternity boyfriends, and several part-time jobs. Brian was just as busy: He attended classes and worked several jobs simultaneously to earn the money needed to pay for tuition, fees, and living expenses – including working nearly every night at the most popular college nightclub in town, The Change of Pace. Neither of us had financial assistance from family, nor did we qualify for grant or scholarship money, so we both worked hard to pay our own way. As an airman in the Illinois Air National Guard at the time, he did receive much of his tuition coverage from the government. But that meant leaving for drill one weekend each month and getting deployed when needed. He was much more grounded than most college guys I knew, and I found I could really count on him, especially in times of crisis.

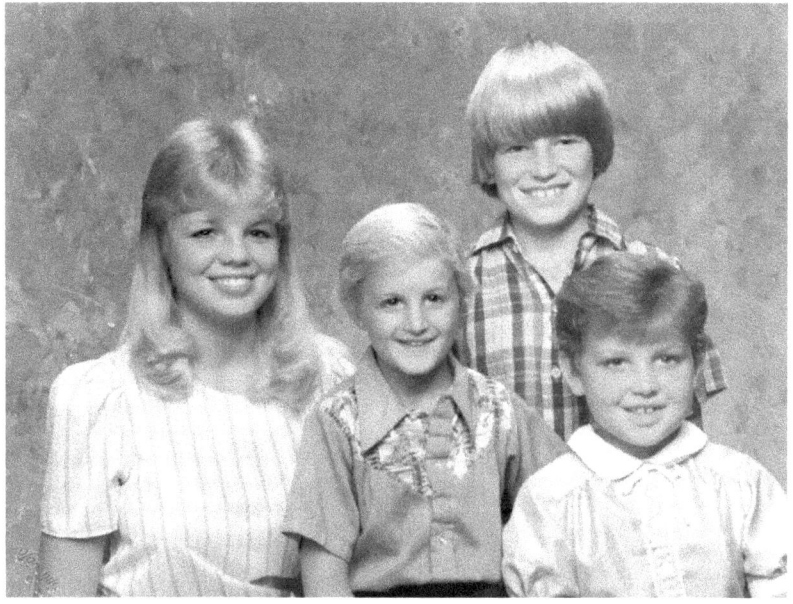

Tammy, Matthew, Brian, and Lyndie

With one semester of classes left before graduation, I made the serious decision to disaffiliate from my sorority. Brian remained one of the few loyal people around me. As much as I loved being a Phi Sigma Sigma, it had become an incredible distraction from my personal goals to graduate on time and begin graduate school the following autumn. After spending the previous three years serving on many committees and on the executive board, I enjoyed having leadership roles, but the commitment had drained me. When I disaffiliated, I was serving as Vice President of Committees,

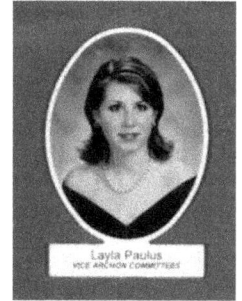

which required time that I did not have since I had to work to pay for school and needed to focus on my grades. In hindsight,

I should have approached my executive board to see how I could take a step back without disaffiliation, but we always seem to have a clearer head after we make certain decisions, don't we?

He was a Christian and I wanted nothing to do with religion at the time. Not having been raised in a church environment like he had been, and being rooted in the sciences, the concept of God just didn't make sense to me. But that did not seem to matter to him, and he would patiently explain when I asked questions about Christianity and about the Bible.

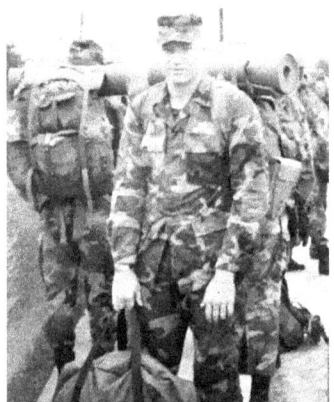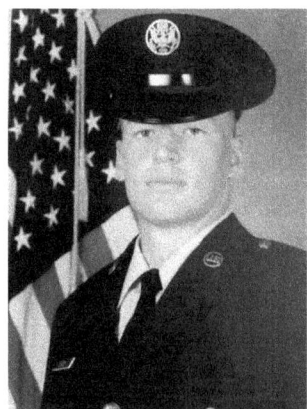

Brian in the US Air Force

Falling in Love

Brian helped me stay focused on the positive things going on in my life when all that I knew had crumbled to ashes that semester. The sorority had defined me the entire time I was a student at WIU, and suddenly, I didn't know who I was without it. Because they took my leaving personally, the girls that had been my constant companions since pledging the sorority years earlier had suddenly become my enemies. I became isolated from all that I knew and struggled with depression as a result. One night outside of the bar where Brian worked, I was involved in a scuffle with a couple of ex-sorority sisters, and before I knew it, he was peeling us all apart. How embarrassing! Brian and I had just begun to explore the idea of dating and there I was in a bar fight with women I had called my sisters only weeks before. When we talk about it to this day, he playfully tells people, "I knew it was love at that moment!"

Brian and I found ourselves spending more time together and our friendship evolved into something much deeper. We became romantically involved and were inseparable that summer in Macomb. Neither of us could stand the idea of being away from the other, and we took advantage of every moment we could spend in each other's company. When we both had time off from work, we would go to the laundromat together, cook meals at his place, work out at the YMCA, or go for a run. Every waking moment—and every sleeping moment, for that matter—we were joined at the hip. At summer's end, after dating for only two months, I left the small college town where we had met and began graduate school in the state's capital city, Springfield, while Brian had two more semesters of classes to complete in Macomb. I was distraught living an hour and a half from him during that first semester of grad school and ended up moving into his apartment with him and his roommate, commuting four days a week for my classes. Our love for one another was extraordinary.

Six months into our cohabitation, I started feeling light-headed and nearly passed out while running at the YMCA one day. Hoping to eliminate the idea of an unplanned pregnancy, I picked up a pregnancy test at Walgreens on my way home. We were blindsided when a purple plus sign appeared in the window of the test.

Having over a year left of graduate school courses and a thesis to work on, I was devastated by the idea of bringing a child into my already chaotic world. In fact, Brian and I had a conversation only days before about my desire not to be a mother and were both in a bit of a funk discovering that we wanted different things in life. I was career-focused, gave no thought to family life, and was a non-believer, while Brian wanted a wife (preferably Christian), children, and to be the breadwinner of his household. But after the initial shock of the news, and many deep conversations about our new development, we both embraced the idea of moving into this new stage of life together.

Telling Our Parents

Once we had time to process all our emotions and discuss our plan to become mom and dad, we were faced with the task of telling our own parents. As was expected, Brian's parents were none too pleased to hear our news.

What *was* surprising, however, was the reaction my mom and dad had when we visited them in my hometown of Monmouth, Illinois. We were nervous because we honestly didn't know what to expect. My parents, though far from perfect, were mostly supportive and genuinely loved Brian even though we had done things in our relationship that were very non-traditional. Not only did we have an intimate relationship out of wedlock, but we had also been living together and sleeping in the same bed every night. My mom was a Christian with a Pentecostal upbringing, while Dad was raised in a large Irish Catholic family, but neither practiced their faith while my brothers and I were growing up, hence my agnostic disposition.

When we approached them in the living room of the house where I had grown up, they were immediately excited, even elated, at the idea of becoming grandparents. My mom seemed relieved because she and I had many combative conversations while I was a teenager about my unwillingness to bear children. She was always disappointed in, and almost ashamed of, my position on motherhood, but her fears had been put to rest. Seeing how excited she was for us to become parents gave me a great sense of pride and put my nerves at ease. I thought, *this really is a beautiful thing, isn't it?* We all hugged and talked about our plans for the future—how I was determined to graduate on time and defend my thesis shortly afterward, and how Brian would support me financially to the best of his ability while we prepared for the baby's arrival. I even brought the book *What to Expect When You're Expecting* so they knew that I was educating myself about what I would experience in the next few months. With my parents in our corner, I felt at ease, and we left their home that day with newfound energy and ambition.

A Roller Coaster of Emotions and a Proposal

We traveled back to the apartment we shared in Macomb that day and made plans to move as soon as the semester ended, since Brian would then be finished with college. Those months were not easy for either of us. I had grown accustomed to going out anytime I wanted, which meant drinking alcohol, much of the time to excess. Now with a growing baby in my belly, that had all ended. Brian continued to work at the bar and I felt very isolated, because all I could do was sit in the apartment alone when I wasn't working. Because in those days everybody still smoked in public places, I quit my job waiting tables at the sports bar where I worked, knowing I didn't want to inhale smoke for eight-hour shifts and risk harming my unborn baby. After I quit, my only source of income was the small amount I received monthly as a graduate assistant, which made my anxiety about money grow exponentially. I was so used to being a go-getter, and this was not what I wanted my life to look like.

Brian and I fought a lot during that time. I was always upset with him for being able to live his life as if nothing had changed, while my life was completely topsy-turvy. Maybe it was pregnancy hormones, but my emotions were always all over the place. I was upset with myself for allowing this pregnancy to happen before being established in a career. We had always been careful, and I was taking my birth control pills like clockwork but still managed to get pregnant. I felt almost betrayed by Brian as he would leave for work and have drinks with his friends, seeming to enjoy life much more than I, and I became consumed with jealousy as Brian's life didn't seem to change at all.

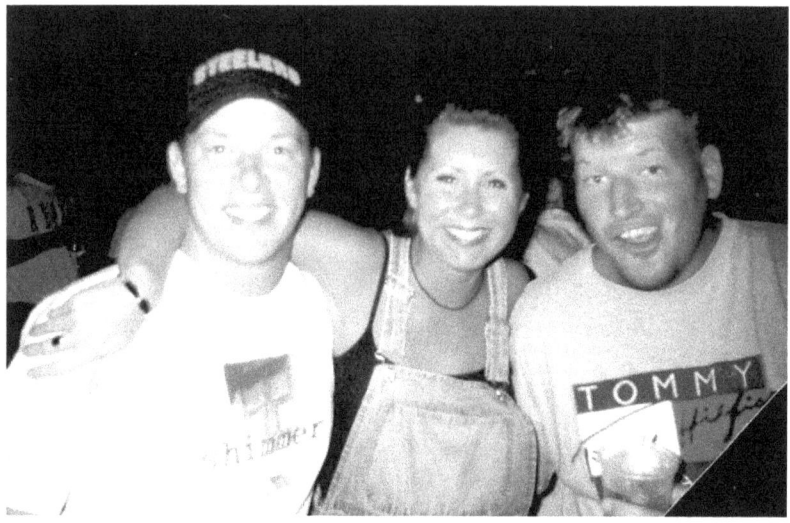

Darrin, me, and Brian

Looking back now, I can see that I was lonely, having lost my friends after dissociating from my sorority, and hurt by my own expectations of what life would look like at the age of 25. I longed for the attention he previously gave me before our lives became complicated. It seemed like every other weekend I was packing up my car to move out and leave him behind. It was such a common occurrence that it actually did become funny! Our other roommate, Darrin, would make jokes about it. He would say, "Hey, are we having a yard sale?" when he saw my things out on the front lawn as I packed them into my little white two-door Chevy Cavalier. We would laugh and I would reply, "Just moving out again!"

But we got through it and grew stronger as partners because, although I did not communicate it well, I discovered just how much I loved Brian and that there was no way in creation that I was willing to do life without him. We had built such a solid foundation by that time in our relationship that it was obvious to not only the two of us, but everyone who knew us, that we were the real deal.

✻

As the semester came to an end and we prepared to leave our college town, Brian surprised me one Saturday morning at our apartment. While I was resting at home from the fatigue that comes along with pregnancy, he was out running errands and picking up breakfast for the two of us. After being gone for a while, he walked through the door with a dozen donuts and a bouquet of the prettiest red roses. Like most ladies, I absolutely loved fresh flowers, but had always told him not to waste money on them since it seemed like a luxury that neither of us could afford. So, when I saw them in his hand, I had a mix of emotions. At first, I thought, *What in the world did you do that for?* but they made me happy, and giving into that happiness, I gave him a big hug for the beautiful sentiment. He set the donuts and roses down in the living room where I sat braless in my pajamas with bedhead and no makeup, then dropped to one knee. He pulled out a small box and opened it, revealing a beautiful glimmer of diamonds and gold, and then asked me to spend the rest of my life with him. I don't know if I had ever been as content as I was at that moment and did not hesitate to say yes. Despite how I looked, I felt beautiful and full of love. We laughed, hugged, and ate donuts as we thought about our future together with our plus one in my belly. Would it be tough? You better believe it! Were we scared out of our minds? You better believe that too! But we were solid, we were fighters, and we were ready for whatever life threw at us.

A new college graduate, Brian decided to move to Springfield while I finished my last year of graduate school. We found a tiny apartment near campus and he began working at a home improvement store earning $10 an hour stocking shelves, while I worked as a graduate assistant for the university's energy studies department chair, earning $700 a month plus a tuition stipend. We were determined to make it work nonetheless, and as uncomfortable as I was with it, I did what I had to do and applied for government assistance during my pregnancy. The Women, Infant, and Children program (WIC) provided my unborn child and me with nutritious food, while the medical card afforded proper health care for both of us. Both programs were a godsend to me, and I used them exactly as they were meant to be used, and once I no longer needed the assistance, I was happy to move on without it.

Welcoming Noah

Being well acquainted with the reality of hard work, I labored feverishly for the next year, finally finishing my coursework in May of 2000.

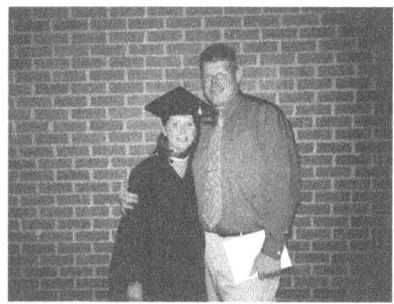 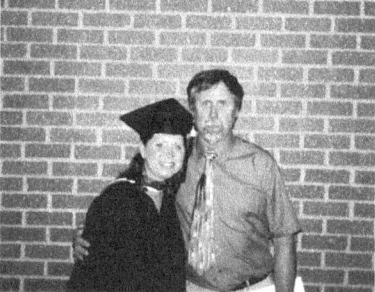

My graduation from UIS. (Left) Me with Brian. (Right) Me with my dad.

I graduated with my master's degree in environmental studies and successfully defended my thesis just in time to welcome our baby boy. My little guy was so comfortable in his momma's belly that my doctor decided to induce labor after we had passed my due date by 10 days. Brian and I arrived at the hospital at 7 a.m. on June 6, 2000. Just like any other day, I prepped with full makeup and beautifully-styled hair, expecting to have a baby in my arms that day—D-day as our military family members knew it. My parents and both of my brothers joined us, and after my water was manually broken, we began the waiting game the best way we all knew how— with lots of laughter and antics from my dad and Brian. But after 17 hours of labor, the laughter had faded, and it was now time to get down to brass tacks.

I pushed for over two hours with very little progression, and when Noah's shoulders had become wedged, my medical team made the decision to transfer me to the operating room while they got scrubbed in. The soon-to-be daddy was handed disposable scrubs that looked like they would be too small for even me, and he took his position next to my head as the cut was made in my lower abdomen. At 12:35 a.m. on June 7, Noah Gerard (named after my dad, Gerard Paul) and I finally became two after an emergency cesarean section, just two years after Brian and I began dating. The overwhelming feeling of love for my nearly nine-pound bundle of joy was like nothing I had ever experienced before that moment. We still tease him because, to this day, that boy is always running late! I have always said, "Noah, you were late for your own birth, and you've been late ever since!" At 24 years old, he doesn't find that quite as funny as the rest of us do.

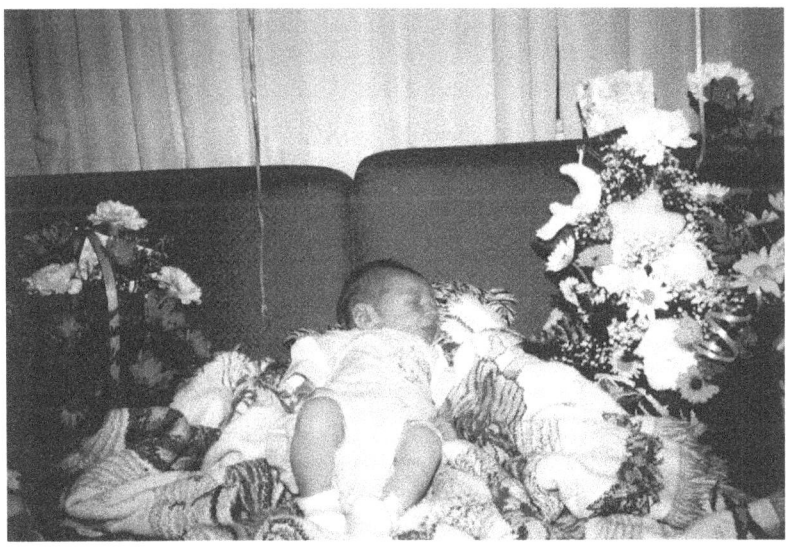

The day we brought Noah home

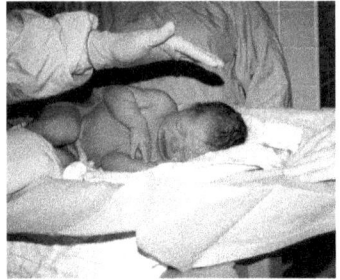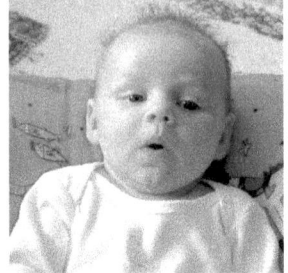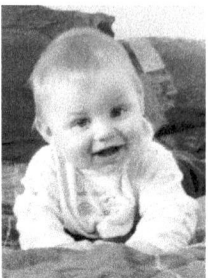

Baby photos of Noah

Shortly after Noah's birth, I began working at a private investigative firm while I was waiting for my big break, so to speak. I simultaneously applied and tested for various positions within government agencies such as the Environmental Protection Agency (EPA) and the Department of Natural Resources (DNR). Working in administration for one of those agencies was my big life dream, and I was determined to make it happen.

By this time, Brian had begun his management career as a trainee in the rental car business. He did so well after completing his training, that he earned his own branch in his hometown of Peoria, cutting our stay in Springfield short. This would be the first time that I would have to put my career dreams and goals on hold for a bit and allow Brian the chance to grow in his career field, but certainly not the last. But that's what motherhood in America looked like, and I was happy to have some time off to be with my baby boy.

Getting Married

Peoria was a fairly typical mid-sized Midwestern city, meant to be only a temporary nest for us. It was surrounded by the same scenery that is indicative of the Midwest: cornfields, livestock pastures, and new housing developments on its perimeter. Being from a small sleepy town, I had my reservations about raising a family there. Although we appreciated much about the city, we felt that if we were not transferred elsewhere soon, it would be better to relocate to the outer suburbs of Peoria and raise our family in a quieter place.

Still unmarried with a toddler, we decided that we really needed to rip the Band-Aid off and finally go through with the ceremony. While Brian was away for training in Florida, I planned our small, cheap wedding that would occur in Las Vegas, enabling his California and Nevada family to be part of it. We had a tight bond with Brian's sister Tammy and her family, and Tammy had become one of my best friends, so we wanted her and her husband Doug to stand up with us. Still having very little disposable income and no outside financial support, our budget was small. Through my research, I found a very afford-able package at the Little White Wedding Chapel and booked flights for Brian, Noah, and me to fly to Vegas, where we would meet up with Tammy, Doug, and their girls, Megan, Chandler, and Alyssa. We stayed at the Aladdin on the strip, where we all swam together the day before our wedding, and had tons of fun, just the eight of us. It felt incredible to be in the company of our biggest supporters and both Brian and I soaked up all the love like two big sponges.

Oh, what a complete mess our wedding day turned out to be! In typical Slater fashion, there was almost nothing that went according to plan. My short hair refused to cooperate in the heat, and my attempt at dramatic smokey eye makeup only ended up making me look like a clown. Thankfully, Tammy was able to help me tame my look a little after I approached Bridezilla status. My glitter dress, which I bought off the rack at Bergner's, was shedding, leaving evidence of my presence everywhere I went. After getting ourselves and our little man ready for the event, Tammy and Doug drove us to get our marriage license, where we were herded through like cattle, while Brian and Tammy's cousin, Corby, looked after all the kiddos. We arrived at the Little White Wedding Chapel pressed for time and were rushed through our 15-minute ceremony in a small room packed with about thirty of Brian's family members.

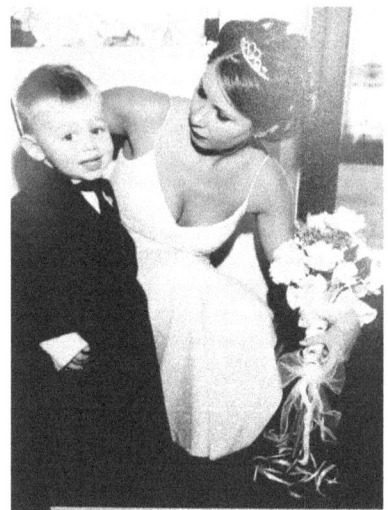 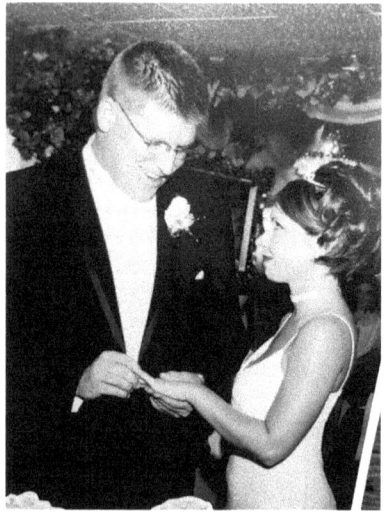

I was so upset by the time I got to the "altar," carrying my 14-month-old son with me, that I barely remember anything about the actual "ceremony." Since my parents did not make the trip to Vegas, I had Noah, all dressed up in his tux, "walk" me down the aisle. Unfortunately, the hem of his little pants had failed, causing him to trip while he walked. Meanwhile, as I would later find out, Brian's mother was outwardly judging my choice to have Noah take that responsibility in my dad's very noticeable absence. My parents had never flown in a plane and couldn't afford the airfare even if they weren't afraid to fly. The air around us, while we were hunkered down in that room, was thick and tense and my face gave way to my emotions, while my ever-content husband-to-be wore his signature smile for all our witnesses and the cameraman.

In no time at all, we were husband and wife, ushered out of there like the place was on fire. On our way out, we were handed a roll of film from the photographer's camera with little more than a "Good luck!" as we all spilled onto the pavement of the parking lot outside. Unbelievable.

I mean, what girl doesn't dream of a wedding like mine? No one, right? Truly, a fairytale beginning to our life of wedded bliss! Little did we know that craziness would continue, and we would really need all the luck we could get.

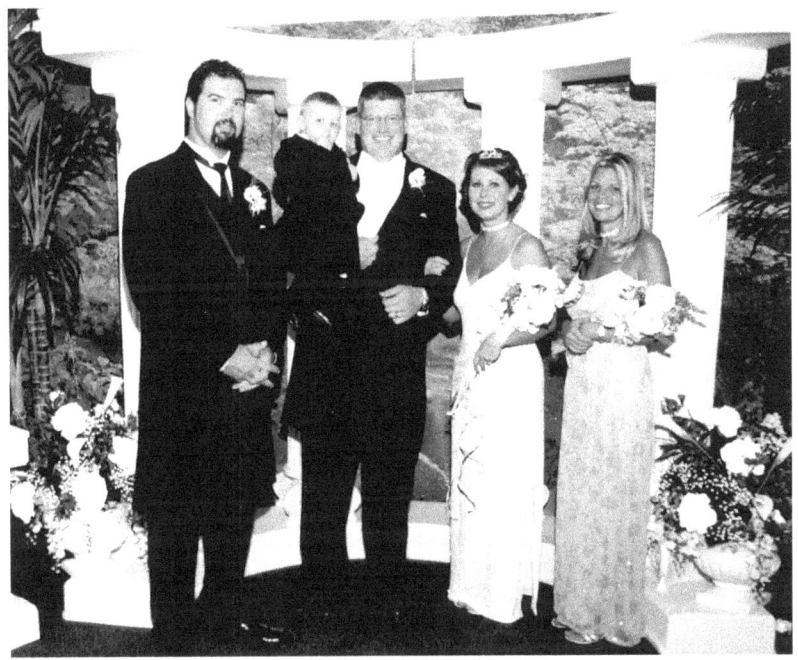

Our wedding party from left to right: Doug, Noah, Brian, me, and Tammy

Once we were home from Vegas, we threw a reception for all our Illinois family and friends so that those who could not fly out to Nevada for our ceremony would feel included. This event went much more smoothly – we reserved a beautiful building in Peoria's warehouse district, the Contemporary Art Center, and cooked our own food to save money (a lot of money, in fact!)

Brian and my dad spent the entire day cooking chicken breasts on the grill outside our small duplex, while Mom and I prepared vegetables and side dishes. We then transported all the food, the cake, and the beverages to the space so by the time the party began, we were all beat! We did what we had to do with a microscopic budget.

It was a lovely evening spent with our greatest friends and family members from all over the state. We danced, laughed, reminisced, and celebrated this new world that we had entered into as a newly married couple with our little boy as the life of the party.

Finding Faith

Back home in Peoria, with the wedding behind us and our bright future as a family ahead of us, I began to truly transform my beliefs in terms of Christianity. We had been attending church where Brian attended services when he lived with his dad. Brian's dad, still uncomfortable with the idea of his son being married to a non-believer, took every opportunity to talk to me about his faith. The conversations that had previously turned me off were now somewhat enlightening, and I became quite engaged. Perhaps it was having a child and bringing a new life into the world that opened my mind to the idea of God. After years of my open-mindedness to Christianity and all it stands for, and digging into the Bible extensively, I decided that I was ready for a relationship with God that I never had before. I wanted to accept Jesus into my heart.

On the floor of the only bathroom in our duplex, I prayed the following prayer of salvation:

> *"Dear Lord, I know that I am a sinner and ask for Your forgiveness. I believe that You died for my sins on the cross and rose from the dead so that I could have eternal life. I invite You to come into my life and wash me of my sins. I trust You and want to follow You as my Lord and Savior. In Jesus' name I pray. Amen."*

On to Nebraska

We were your typical young, middle-class, Midwestern American family. Brian and I both had bachelor's degrees and I had a master's degree. We were following our dreams of nailing down great careers with remarkable companies where we could continue to climb the metaphorical ladder. We both had respectable jobs for the time being, but also had bigger aspirations. He was managing his own store for a major car rental company, and I landed a position for a local health department in the field of environmental health. We were on our way to the 2.2 children, white-picket-fence American dream, especially since we were now married and expecting another baby within a few months.

Brian was promoted within the car rental company and received a salary increase with great commission potential, so we again prepared to move to another city. He became branch manager of the second largest store in Nebraska, located in downtown Lincoln, and though we knew not a soul there, we embraced the move as a great opportunity.

Noah, now two and a half, was eagerly anticipating the arrival of his new sibling in a few short months, and life was full of promise for all of us. We packed up our small, single-level Peoria duplex into a U-Haul truck, fastened our only vehicle to its hitch, kissed our families goodbye, and headed out of town.

Having an environmental science background, I soon became employed with a federal government agency under the umbrella of the United States Department of Agriculture (USDA) called the Natural Resources Conservation Service (NRCS)—a dream come true for me. The possibilities for upward mobility within the agency were endless and I truly felt that we were finally where we were destined to be.

We took on our new roles as Husker fans in the "Land of Red" and enjoyed exploring our new surroundings. Since we have always delighted in attending sporting events, we took in an occasional baseball game, and we frequented the downtown eateries and shops. Our three-level town home was set in a lovely neighborhood that was centrally located. We took advantage of the walking/biking trail that wound through our backyard by taking family walks nearly every evening after work. We all seemed to fit right into this new life. Lincoln was such a beautiful city, and we were truly at peace with this move, planning to make it our final destination.

Though we had no family in Nebraska, it did not take us long to make a flock of friends. Brian and I both worked with friendly folks who were eager to help and had a genuine interest in our family. Though most of my coworkers lived in or around Wahoo (35 minutes away), we tried to meet up occasionally for a night out. I had never really experienced such a solid connection with new people in my life as I did while we lived in Nebraska.

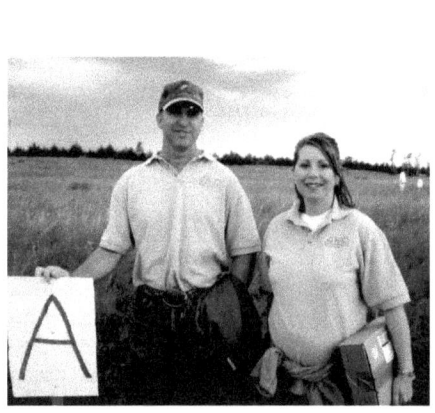

In the field with NRCS

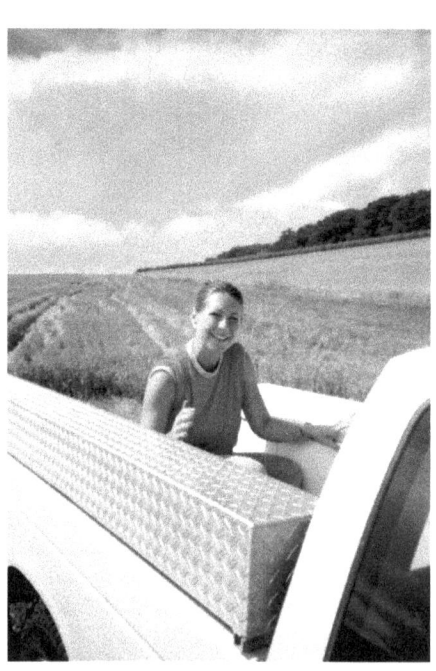

Even while we made our evening journeys on the trail, most walkers who passed by acknowledged us with a smile and a "hello." Initially, I remember feeling struck in a sort of odd way as this was unusual behavior in my past world. I found it refreshing and peaceful, and to this day wonder what life would be like if we still lived in Nebraska.

CHAPTER THREE

The ICU Giant and Her Invalid Mother

ABIGAIL GRACE WAS BORN AT 11:42 a.m., weighing 4 pounds, 15 ounces and measuring 17.5 inches long. According to the doctors' notes during her birth, she had no heart tone, no spontaneous respiration, and no detectable heart rate. In layperson's terms, Abigail was not alive at birth.

Apgar

Before I tell you about Abigail's Apgar scores, let's take a moment to learn about the Apgar test to really take in how dire Abigail's situation was at birth. According to the American Baby & Child Law Centers:

> The Apgar test is an assessment of a newborn baby's vital signs that is a quick indication to the delivery team of the health of the child. A rating system is used for each letter in the acronym that is added up where a score of anywhere from 7 to 10 represents a healthy newborn baby.
>
> The A in Apgar represents the skin color of the infant. A healthy baby will display an allover pink color, accounting for a 2, while anything less than pink accounts for a 0 or a 1.

The P represents the baby's heart rate. An absent heartbeat earns the baby a 0, a rate of less than 100 beats a minute (bpm) will score a 1, and anything over 100 bpm will score a 2.

The G is the baby's reflex response, and the score is based on the baby's "grimace" as they respond to stimulation. No response merits a 0, grimacing ears a 1, and crying or screaming scores a 2. Muscle tone is represented by the second A in Apgar and is rated from limp to some movement, to active motion, again rated with a 1, 2, or 3 respectively.

And finally, the R represents the baby's breathing ability. If the baby is not breathing at birth, they earn a 0, barely breathing is a 1, and breathing well is a 2.

The scores are added up at one minute after birth, then at five minutes, and finally at ten minutes.

With Abigail's score total starting at 0 in the first-minute assessment, improving to 4 at five minutes, and finally reaching five at the 10-minute assessment, we can come to our own conclusion that she was far from healthy after her arrival into our world. She was revived by bag-mask ventilation and chest compressions and was finally intubated. Still, in the first ten minutes of her life, Abigail showed extremely poor tone, responsiveness, and serious discoloration. She was immediately given the first of countless IVs, which would eventually lead to a central venous catheter (PICC line) being surgically implanted. The team placed her on mechanical ventilation and prepared her for transport for the five-minute drive to a third hospital, St. Elizabeth of Lincoln. Although she was stabilized by oxygen and ventilation, there was no doubt in the minds of those on her medical team that Bryan LGH did not have the facilities to manage such a touchy case.

Completely incoherent during the delivery of my battered

baby girl, I unfortunately do not remember a single detail of her birth. Because I had my own physical issues to which medical personnel needed to attend, I was robbed of the joy that a mother hopes to feel associated with the birth of her only little girl.

Because I was unconscious, not in labor, and time was not on our side due to the baby's condition, the doctors were forced to make an incision from my belly button to my pubic bone to deliver her via emergency cesarean section. It was a barbaric method but necessary to ensure the survival of my unborn child.

To shed further light on my condition, my pelvis was fractured on both the right and left sides, which accounted for the worst of my pain. My entire right side was battered from the impact of the second truck that T-boned my car, accounting for the secondary pain that I felt. The tissue in my right wrist, rotator cuff, and breast absorbed much of the second impact. Having no memory of my daughter's birth, I learned about the procedure from my husband and later by reading through reams of medical records. Even now, more than 20+ years later, I deal with the pain daily.

Brian's Strength

Brian recalls that he followed the transporters around from one hospital to the next, whether it was by helicopter or ambulance, like a lost puppy. Sick with worry, he was rarely informed any more than I because of the sheer delicacy of the situation. All parties involved were focused solely on Abigail's and my well-being, and time was of the essence. Thank God for Brian's coworker, who chauffeured him from hospital to hospital, as I cannot even imagine him driving in such an emotional state. But as always, my cast-iron husband held all the pieces together.

Arriving at Bryan LGH, he discovered that the baby would be delivered but he would not be allowed to join the team during delivery. Many fathers want to be just as involved in the process of their child's first breath as mothers are, which made it heartbreaking for me to know that he was also robbed of such a precious opportunity.

Because I was still unconscious when Abigail was being hastily transferred to yet another hospital, Brian was the first to learn the baby's gender. Once Abigail was stabilized, the doctor appeared in the waiting room where my husband was pacing around in anticipation of some news. The doctor simply told Brian that the child was born and would immediately be transported to St. Elizabeth Hospital. In all the bustle and confusion, Brian didn't think to ask whether we were the new parents of a boy or a girl until his coworker, Ron, spoke up. "Hey," he leaned toward Brian in curiosity, "was it a boy or a girl?" Brian then rushed after the doctor. "Hey, Doc, boy or girl?" he shouted. "It's a girl!" the doctor exclaimed as he threw his celebratory arms into the air and rushed in the opposite direction.

A bundle of nerves, the 6'3", 280-pound new daddy returned to playing the hurry-up-and-wait game. Meanwhile, the team of experts hastened behind the scenes to get our fragile baby girl prepared for the transport to her newest temporary home at St. Elizabeth Hospital. Before long, she was abruptly escorted through the hospital corridors in her Isolette by a team of medical personnel. They found their way to the waiting area and quickly presented Abigail to her daddy, unable to be touched or held. The tiny creature with coal-black hair and big blue eyes lay surrounded by a bubble of plastic and cords attached to machines that were her lifeline and would be for months to come. There was only time for a quick introduction between Daddy and daughter, and they were off again, making their way to the ambulance waiting just outside.

For the next five days, my husband was in two places at once. Because of the severity of my injuries, I called Bryan LGH my home during this time, while Abigail was fighting for her life in one hospital after another. As if it were not enough that my injuries caused by the impact of the accident itself were severe, I now had new incisions that were a result of my emergency cesarean section. Not exactly the kind of scar that a 28-year-old woman hopes to bear for the rest of her life, but it was a necessary evil.

Frantic on the inside, yet somehow calm on the exterior, Brian followed Abigail and her medical team to St. Elizabeth Hospital just a few minutes away, since they would undoubtedly need parental consent for more tests and procedures. Meanwhile, I was slowly coming back to reality and quickly found that I much preferred to go back to being unconscious. The pain was the most horrific that I had ever felt, and I nearly wore out the button connected to the machine that delivered morphine to my veins over the next few days. Amid all the chaos, Brian managed to call family and friends and tell them an abridged version of what had happened that day.

My parents, Gerry and Denice, were the most difficult to locate since they were not yet hip to the idea of cell phones, and they were both at work at the time of the accident. Working as a phlebotomist on a blood drive that day, my mom could not be reached, and my dad worked on a forklift, making it nearly impossible to reach him as well. My poor husband was tasked with hunting them both down by any means necessary to deliver the horrific news. To locate my mom, he had to first call the blood donation company for which she worked and find out where the blood drive was taking place.

After getting the phone number of one of her field managers, he hastily dialed in hopes of connecting with Mom. The same occurred as he attempted to locate Dad: he had to call the main office of Butler Manufacturing in Galesburg, Illinois, and have them page him—no easy feat. The steel yard where Dad spent his weekdays was quite extensive, and his foreman was tasked with getting a message to Dad to call Brian.

After they were finally located, Brian had to craftily articulate the severity of the situation without sending my parents into a frenzy, since they had a six-and-a-half-hour drive ahead of them. Hearing the news, they were understandably frantic, but somehow made the drive to Nebraska, wasting no time. After arriving, they stayed by my bedside for several days, and afterward my dad commuted back and forth to see Abigail, just as Brian did.

The First NICU Experience

While Abigail was housed at St. Elizabeth, her medical team was taken aback by some alarming findings. Initially, the reports were simply that she had a soft anterior fontanelle, but that was before she was stable enough from a cardiac standpoint for more stringent tests to be performed. Upon reexamination, it was found that the soft spot on the right parietal area of the skull was found to warrant a complete skull series.

These findings showed that she indeed suffered a skull fracture, bringing the pediatric neurosurgeons promptly to the scene. She underwent a CT scan to see a more detailed account of the happenings inside her tiny, premature head. It was discovered that the skull fracture crossed the sagittal sinus (the vein that travels over the top part of the head) and there was intraventricular (occurring inside the ventricles of the brain) and posterior occipital bleeding (subsequent bleeding in the lower back part of the brain).

A chest x-ray showed what they called mild-to-moderate hyaline membrane disease and respiratory distress syndrome (RDS). Even without understanding all the medical jargon, this was obviously a serious matter. To the medical personnel on the case, it was even more serious than they could withstand at St. Elizabeth. The next move was to the Children's Hospital in Omaha, and it would be immediate. Still on a ventilator and stuffed to the gills with Phenobarbital, an anti-seizure medication, my tiny baby girl was again transported via ambulance, this time to endure the 60-mile journey to Omaha.

Abigail reached her destination, the Neonatal Intensive Care Unit (NICU) at the Children's Hospital in Omaha, late into the night on the day of her birth. There was a team of specialists waiting for her once again, and she was intubated and placed on a ventilator promptly. Once they were able to delve into her case, they found further cause for alarm. In broad terms, she had what they called a traumatic cranial cerebral injury, which was a considerably basic method of describing what I only learned years after the episode. A CT scan ordered by the pediatric neurosurgeon showed that she had blood in the lateral, third, and fourth ventricles of her brain. In medical terms, she had an *intraventricular hemorrhage, bilateral posterior interhemispheric hemorrhage, subdural acute hemorrhages, and subarachnoid hemorrhages*; in terms the rest of us can understand, she had severe brain bleeds in several regions of her brain. As if this were not a tall enough hurdle for the tiny girl to overcome, *a vertical and transverse skull fracture was found in the right parietal area.*

Given the fact that she was eight weeks premature, Abigail had plenty of catching up to do developmentally, even without the injuries. Although babies who are born during the beginning of the eighth month have a great chance for survival, it is within the last two months of pregnancy that the brain grows and matures substantially. Since most of her injuries were sustained on her brain, the odds were doubly stacked against her. Her lungs had also not yet developed to their fullest potential, forcing her to become quite acquainted with the ventilator over the next several weeks.

During her stay in the Children's Hospital NICU, Room 470, she underwent one intrusive test after another, received several blood transfusions, and had an endless number of IVs placed before finally having a central line inserted. Her tiny veins just could not withstand the IVs and would collapse so the central line would bypass the veins altogether. It was safer and more secure, avoiding repeated needle sticks by administering all medication through a single line. She underwent one brain surgery and then another, while her father and I could do nothing more than sit by her side patiently, watch in horror, and pray constantly.

Brian had no choice but to travel an hour each way from Lincoln to Omaha, and then back again daily, while I remained at Bryan LGH. He would stay with me during the days while I was mostly awake, and as soon as I slept at night, he would make the long drive over to Abigail's bedside until he could no longer hold his eyes open. Then he would groggily travel back to Lincoln where he might or might not sleep, only to do it all again the next morning. It's a miracle that he never fell asleep behind the wheel as exhausted as he was all the time.

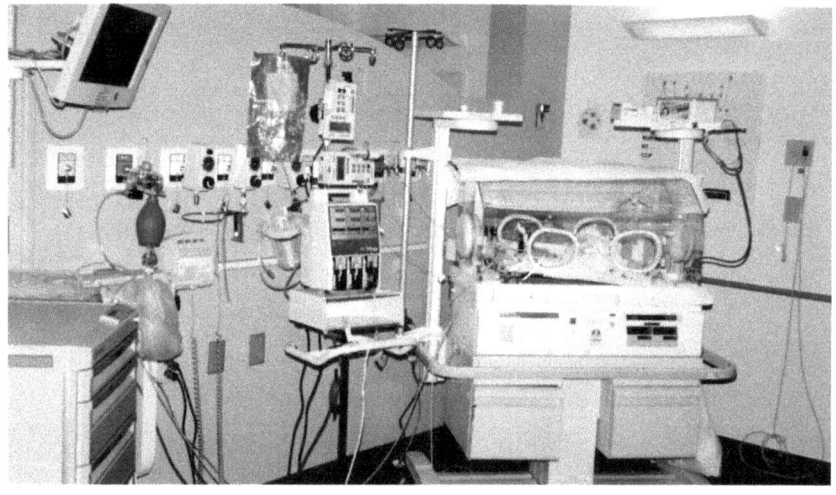

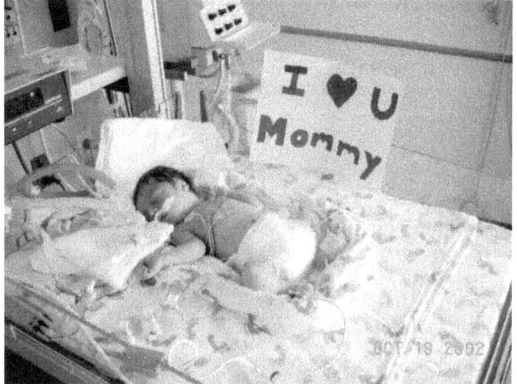

Abi in her Isolette with the machines that kept her alive

My Baby in Pictures

While Brian sat by Abigail's side, he took photos of her to bring to me in the mornings. This, aside from the enormous carving on my torso, was the only evidence I had of my new baby's existence. I had not been able to see her in the flesh, hold her, or to hear her cry.

He did warn me before showing me the photos that it would be heavy for me to see, and he was right. It broke my heart into pieces to see her tiny, bloated body hooked up to several machines. She was unable to breathe, excrete waste, or eat on her own. Imagine what that was like! It was as if she were a machine herself. She had a tube coming out of her nose that fed her, and a tube coming out of her mouth that breathed life into her. There were many colorful lines attached to her chest, each having its own duty to perform. Every line led to a monitor that told the nursing staff what her vital signs were at all times. Any time one of the vital signs dropped below or escalated above normal, alarms would sound to notify the nurse of a problem. Her foot was wrapped in a cuff, as was her tiny wrist—these were to monitor blood pressure and oxygen levels.

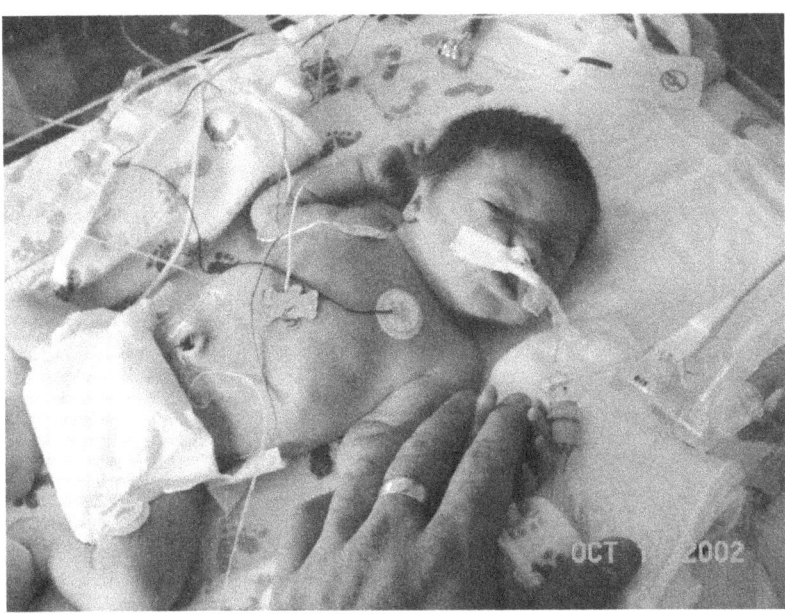

There was one particular photo that my dad took of Brian's hand next to Abigail's body that put into perspective exactly how miniature she was, even though she was a giant compared to all her preemie NICU neighbors. What struck me, especially in this photo, was that it seemed his wedding band could have fit around her wrist. I was awestruck and terrified for her, and I wanted nothing more than to meet her. This was my goal. I had to get out of that depressing bed and show the doctors and therapists that I was ready to be on my own. Until I was able to meet her, I was trapped inside the walls of my own "prison."

Those sweet, heartbreaking photos meant everything to me and gave me a reason to fight through my own pain. As difficult as some of those photos were to see, I am, and forever will be, grateful for that gift from my husband and the early connection they provided.

My Own Healing Continued

For the next five days, I endured an exhausting number of treatments to get me healthy enough to check out of Bryan LGH. Because I had a collapsed lung, the therapists would come into my room every few hours to help me restore its maximum breathing capacity. To sort of "reinflate" the lung, I had to suck in air using a spirometer as hard as I could inhale, and then force the air back out of the lungs hard and fast. They were such an inconvenience! I hated to see those people walk through the door because I knew how hard I would have to work while they were there. When we are healthy, we take so much for granted. Who would have thought that it could be this difficult to breathe?

One of the worst things about my recovery was the large gash that was now a permanent part of my midsection. Since the surgery was performed in an emergency, I was stitched back together like a junior high home economics project.

Uneven and thick, the suture was hideous and mimicked drapery hanging from a window. More importantly, it was almost as painful as the fractured pelvis. It hurt to laugh, cry, cough, sneeze, and sit up—yet another example of activities we inevitably take for granted when we are healthy.

I was somewhat familiar with this type of pain since Noah was delivered via C-section, but that was through what they called a "bikini cut" incision. It in no way prepared me for the pain of an incision that was four times the size and extended through many of my abdominal muscles. The pain from this split in my gut was one that lingered far longer than I hoped.

The worst part of my hospital stay was rolling over onto my side. Again, another thing we take for granted when we have healthy, unfractured bones. The nurses and therapists would "log roll" me so I would not get too comfortable lying on my back (or as they explained, it kept me from getting bedsores and stiffness). Every time they did this it was like breaking my hip all over again. The log roll involved several nurses moving me with a blanket that was situated beneath me. With each tug, I would cry and scream in agony.

My Loving Support System

My mom, a licensed nurse, was usually there to place the pillows where they needed to go. I would need several at my back, one between my legs, two under my arms, and two at my feet. These would keep my pelvis aligned, removing undue pressure on my fractures. Since I had one fracture on the left side pubic area and one on my right back side, this became a tricky game that never really worked out perfectly. I would hear the most awful crackling noises coming from my pelvis and the pain was almost unbearable. "Log roll" would forever be a hauntingly painful cluster of words for me to hear. "Layla," one of the nurses would say, "it's time to roll over onto your side." I would ask for just a few minutes to load my veins up with morphine by tapping the red button that delivered it through the IV. They never argued. Even so, I could not suffer through a log roll without weeping.

My parents were available as much as they could be, considering that they lived two states away and had jobs from which they could not be away from for long. While in Lincoln, Mom mostly stayed with me in my room, while Dad traveled back and forth between the two hospitals, much like Brian did. Dad developed a bond with Abi right away, and being a daddy's girl myself, I perfectly understood her attachment to him. She recognized his kind voice and would use all her might to attempt to gaze in his direction as he softly talked to her.

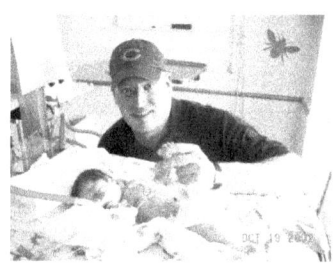

Brian with Abi

Besides the frequent visits from her daddy and grandpa, I am convinced that God was ever present in her life from the second she transformed from a fetus into a baby. I picture Him holding her undersized hand and soothing her with His mighty, yet gentle voice during the times when she was otherwise alone in her Isolette. I believe she was fortunate enough to develop a relationship with Him that those of us who have never suffered in such a way could ever understand. It was that soothing voice and delicate touch that no one else could provide but Him which eased her into every new day; of that I am certain.

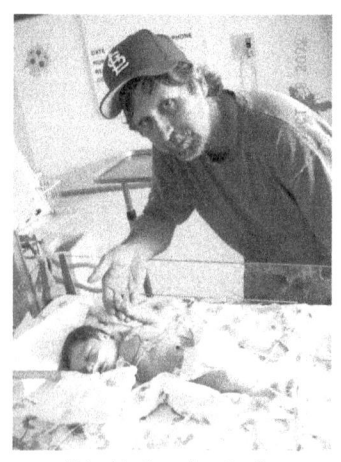

Abi with Grandpa Paulus

While Abigail was in Children's Hospital, I began to pump and store my milk so that she could "drink" it through her feeding tube. This was a difficult and painful task because of the bruising and swelling on my entire right side. The milk in my right breast was arduous coming in because the milk ducts were terribly swollen and clogged with blood. This meant I had to manually extract the milk by methodically massaging my breast. I hope it suffices to say that this was not a painless process. Using the breast pump was a stressful experience and I loathed it nearly as much as I loathed lying in bed. I stored the milk in containers, the nurses froze it, and Brian transported it to Abigail every night when he left to visit her.

Since my medical providers were well aware of the disastrous situation in which my family and I were involved, we informally came to an agreement about a plan to get me out of my hospital bed. I worked laboriously to become well enough to leave the security of doctors, nurses, therapists, and equipment and dive into new, unchartered waters at Children's Hospital. A discharge summary reads as follows:

> *The patient would like to go to Omaha to be closer to her baby. She will stay at the Rainbow House. She will attend outpatient physical therapy at Methodist Hospital. She has full weight bearing on the left leg, 20 pounds weight bearing on the right leg. She will need to use a walker. She may shower. Staples were removed from her abdominal incision. Steri-strips placed. No lifting more than 10 to 15 pounds. No driving until seen by orthopedics. . .*

Using the Walker

Ah, the walker. It would be my independence and my enemy simultaneously. It was what stood between me and my baby for days. As part of our informal plan, my physical therapist reported that I would only be released from my stay at Bryan LGH when I could climb the hallway stairs independently, with only my walker to use for assistance. My will was not to be underestimated.

I began using my walker to do things like go to the bathroom alone. This led to walking the halls of the hospital every chance I had, and soon I was attempting those stairs to which the therapist referred. Through a waterfall of tears, I would stand at the bottom, inspecting the mountain that stood between me and my freedom from this place. Battling that first step was such a painful struggle that I knew it would be no easy feat. Standing on one step with my walker on the one above it to keep me steady, I would go up and down only two or three steps at a time. I was winded easily, having only partial lung capacity, and because of the insufferable pain in both of my fractured hips, it took everything I had to step up. But I was determined to conquer what had become my very own Mount Everest. The next time I was allowed to walk with my new wheeled walker, I would go a bit further (only after maxing out my morphine dosage on my pain pump, of course). Although it took a few days to do it, I finally accomplished the hellish goal that my therapist set for me. Even after I was totally doped up, I cried all the way up and all the way down that mountain from the sheer pain, but it was worth every tear. In a short time I would be headed to NICU, Room 470, at Children's Hospital of Omaha, and not a second too soon.

My progress was only just beginning, and I had a long, strenuous road ahead of me but, with the permission of my medical team, I was elated to check out of that hospital five days after being admitted. There were strings attached, of course, and I had to promise to participate in daily physical therapy while in Omaha. It worked out quite nicely since therapy was only a hop, skip, and a jump (or for me, a long, treacherous, painful scoot) from Abi's room. It became part of my daily routine and helped me keep motivated to get stronger with time so that I could hold my new baby girl when the opportunity finally arose. The therapy would last from October 23 until November 29, when I was released from my outpatient recovery responsibilities.

While I was tackling Mt. Everest at Bryan LGH, Abigail was struggling to do the same in Omaha. It seemed that every day brought with it more disturbing news. I could hardly deal with being away from her and knowing of her progress, or lack thereof, only by way of reports. I learned that she was finally diagnosed with the following:

> *Intraventricular hemorrhage, subdural hematoma, subarachnoid hemorrhages, perinatal asphyxia, skull fracture, hyaline membrane disease, possible sepsis, 32-week gestation prematurity and placental abruption at birth.*

Not knowing medical jargon, this all sounded absolutely hopeless to me, but I knew one thing with no doubt in my heart: I knew that God was not a cruel God, and that He would never have let Abigail survive the impact of the accident just to let her fade in an incubator at a hospital. That belief kept me in a constructive mindset, and I had faith that God would lead her through all of this with the least amount of pain possible.

Meeting Abigail

October 23, 2002, was a triumphant day—it was the day I met my tiny daughter. I stumbled into her NICU room late that night, courtesy of my mother and, ironically, a red two-door rental car, not unlike my own car which had been destroyed weeks earlier. She chauffeured Noah and me from Lincoln to Omaha, where Brian awaited our arrival. The moment was glorious and flawed, but it was all mine. I can only imagine what people thought of me as I made my way across the NICU floor with my steel-wheeled companion assisting me. I was thirty-two shades of black and blue from head to foot on my right side and tears plunged down my cheeks as I pushed my way through the otherwise quiet corridors. My front teeth were chipped from the collision, and I had various cuts and scrapes on my face. Nonetheless, I knew that none of this would matter to my newborn who lay in her Isolette, waiting to meet the woman responsible for this mess we were in.

My tiny, dark-haired angel was beyond beautiful to me. At

nearly five pounds, she far outweighed many of her newborn neighbors, some of whom weighed as little as one and a half pounds. I was in awe of the machines, monitors, tubes, and wires that were working overtime to keep her alive. The situation appeared fragile, yet incredible at the same time. Every function that her body performed was accounted for on the monitors that hung on the walls. Her breathing, blood oxygen levels, blood pressure, and heart rate were all things that were closely examined every second of the day. By this time, she had become less swollen and had lost a bit of weight compared to her birth weight, mostly because she was so bloated with fluids. She was upgraded from a table to an Isolette after finishing her UV light treatments, which were administered to improve her jaundiced skin. This table resembled a baby cot but was not enclosed like the Isolette. They cocooned her by swaddling her and placing rolled blankets all around her body to secure her. Because the doctors felt confident that she would be able to breathe on her own and urinate regularly, this was also the day she was taken off the ventilator and her Foley catheter was removed.

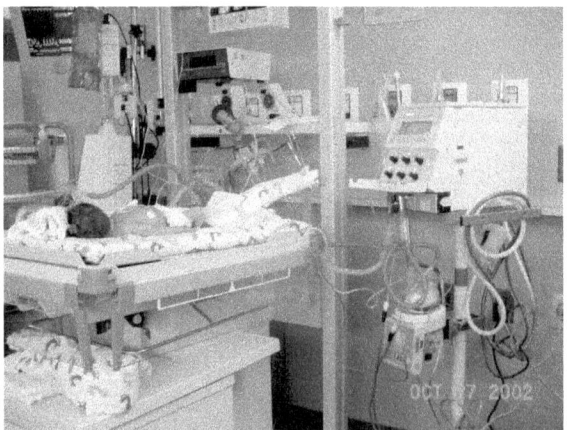

Brian and I chose to believe God and not necessarily the doctors who were specialists in her case. We would continue in good faith that the Lord would lead us to a partial understanding of what His plan was for Abigail, as well as for our family. There were many times that the doctors would tell us of her prognosis, and it was bleak at best. I remember one specific instance where, after being out of the hospital for only a week myself, one of the neonatologists pulled up a chair to discuss Abi's future with us. There was a sort of joke among the NICU parents about your child's doctor pulling a chair over. You did not want to see them sit down in your child's room because you knew it was not going to be good news.

This proved to be the case for us. He began to speak in all this medical mumbo-jumbo, for lack of a better description, and none of it really made sense to us. After listening to the doctor respectfully, Brian finally asked a simple question that came with a devastating answer. "What does all of this mean?" he asked. "Is she ever going to be normal?" After what seemed like an eternal pause, the doctor answered. He told us, in his typical medical matter-of-fact way, that the likelihood of Abigail ever being "normal" was slim. He proceeded to explain to us that she could end up in a variety of different states, varying from mild cerebral palsy to total vegetation. Neither of us could believe what we were hearing. We immediately broke down, weeping in each other's arms. This was the first time since the accident occurred that I saw my husband give in to his emotions. We were absolutely devastated and, for the time being, hopeless.

The next several days brought some major accomplishments and we were temporarily able to celebrate. On October 24, Abigail was taken off oxygen, lost her belly IVs, and began "drinking" breast milk. On October 28, we were able to give her a bath for the first time and finally hold her. Eleven whole days since she had been born and I was finally able to hold my little angel in my arms! The only way she could be touched prior to this day was softly with a finger, preferably a gloved one. Her skin was delicate, almost translucent, and so fragile that we were limited to minimal physical contact with her until this day. It was a torturous situation for us as her parents, but also for her as a newborn who needed to be touched and cuddled. We had another celebration on that day: at 7:00 p.m., Abigail was moved to a crib of her own.

The following day, Abigail was moved up to 6 cc (1 cc, or cubic centimeter, is smaller than a teaspoon – just a few drops, really) of breast milk an hour through her tube. Before this, she had been taking only three to four. Small steps forward were much preferred to backward movement. I was also able to hold her again, making October 28 and 29 two of the most important days in her progress so far. We were elated, but still cautious.

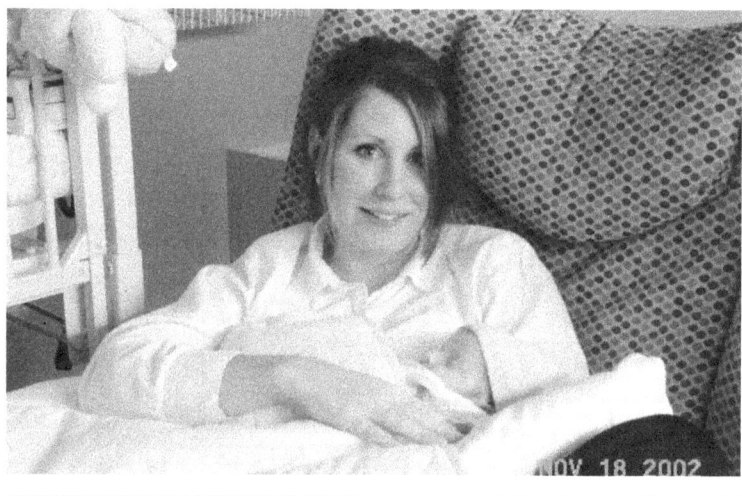

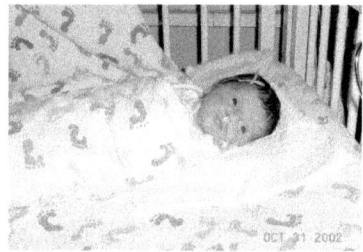
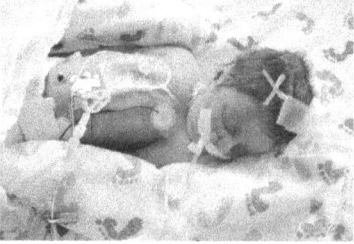

One worry that lingered in our minds during these triumphant days was that the doctors continued performing ultrasounds of her head to keep close tabs on the ventricles in her brain. Her ventricles progressively increased in size, which meant they were filling up with fluid as time progressed. The hope was that we would eventually see this fluid build-up diminish.

The Explanation

The reason for the ventricular expansion was that Abigail's body was not draining the cerebrospinal fluid from around her brain the way that it naturally should. Instead, the fluid was finding crevices to flow into, which were precisely what the ventricles became. This essentially is a description for yet another medical term, hydrocephalus, which was added to the already exhaustive list of ailments. As her head continued to swell, the doctors warned us that the need for surgical intervention would likely come soon. This meant placing a device called a shunt into her ventricle to mechanically drain the cerebrospinal fluid from her ever-expanding brain.

Faith Grows

I don't recall praying so much in my life as I did during this time, nor do I think I have prayed as hard since. As a mother, it was devastating to imagine my daughter's already fragile skull being opened to have some foreign object surgically placed inside her miniature brain. The many chats I had with my pastor back home in Illinois humbled me, but they didn't force me to change my tactics at the time. When I asked him "why me?" his blunt reply was, "Why *not* you? Do you somehow think you are different from the rest of us? Bad things happen to good people all the time." Ouch! As much as that stung, it has stayed with me since and I think of that conversation every time I ask myself, "Why is this happening to me?" Now, I ask instead, "What can I learn from this?" and "How is this helping me grow?"

I begged and pleaded with God all day, every day. "Please Lord, I pray You will allow me to witness for myself an extraordinary miracle that only You can perform. I pray that the fluid will miraculously drain on its own to avoid such an intense medical procedure on my sweet baby girl. Please, Lord, I beg of You, perform this miracle for me and I shall never cease in my efforts to give all glory to You. In Jesus' name, Amen."

And as the days crept by with no miracle in sight, I became so desperate that I found myself bargaining with God, almost bullying Him to make things go my way, not His.

This desperation grew and my promises and tactics became all the more exaggerated when I felt He was not listening to me. "The Bible says, 'Ask and you shall receive,' and 'You have not because you ask not.'" I would throw His own words back into His face expecting that He would surely grant me this wish, right? As if He were a genie in a bottle. "Why are You doing this to me? I have been taught that you will never forsake me, and yet. . ."

But God doesn't work that way, does He? Sometimes we have to suffer through the worst parts to know when we are experiencing the beautiful parts. And as much as we beg, plead, threaten, question, and beg some more, EVERYTHING works out according to His plan and in His perfect timing. Always. We just have to be patient and let God do the work for us.

To learn more about the medical terms and topics discussed in this chapter, visit this link:

www.SavingAbigailGrace.com

CHAPTER FOUR

The Carolyn Scott Rainbow House

WE MOVED INTO THE CAROLYN Scott Rainbow House the night that I was released from my own medical "prison." A beautifully cared-for three-story brick dwelling, the Rainbow House was a home away from home for families of patients at Children's Hospital of Omaha for a small nightly cost. This was our home from October 23, 2002, through December 1, 2002. I was fortunate enough to stay in a first-floor handicap-accessible room, equipped with a bathroom specially designed for those with limitations such as mine. We had two double beds in the room as well, allowing Brian, Noah, and me to live comfortably, since we did not spend much time there together. Mom stayed with us in Noah's bed for a few days after we arrived, giving us the freedom to come and go from Abi's room together without having to worry about Noah's care. My mom's assistance during those days was invaluable and deeply appreciated.

The first several weeks of Abi's life were wearisome, but we soon developed a routine and a sense of normalcy. Our days consisted of waking early so that one of us could be in her NICU room when the doctors made their rounds. That meant that we needed to be there between 7:00 and 8:00 a.m. in hopes of learning new information. Once Mom went back to Illinois, we were forced to take turns doing this so that one of us could take care of Noah at the Rainbow House. We were careful to make sure Noah stayed on a schedule and never felt that he was being overlooked. Usually, I would take the day shift with Abi, and Brian would take over after dinner, sometimes staying until 3:00 or 4:00 a.m. We wanted to be sure that she was only without one of her parents for the smallest amount of time possible. When Mom was not with us, Brian had to wake Noah and bundle him up to drive me to the hospital since I was not able to drive for eight weeks after the accident.

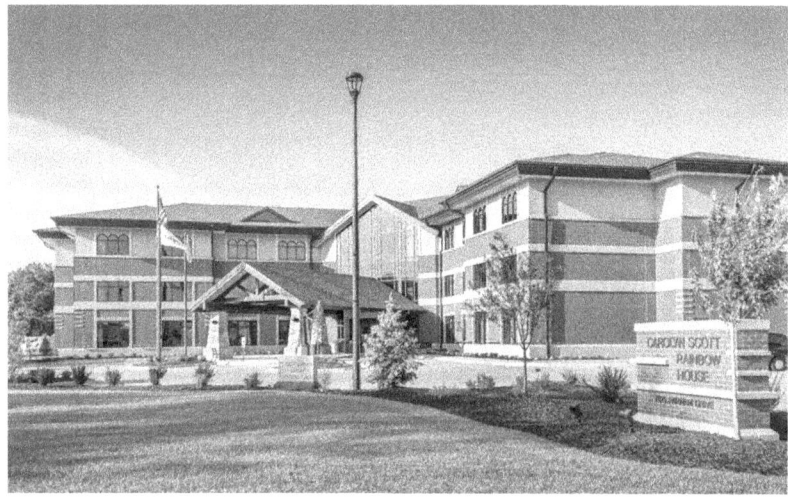

I stopped at the hospital coffee shop to get a mocha nearly every morning to sip on while I read my Bible and watched Abi sleep. As soon as she woke, I rushed over (as quickly as I could with my walking companion) and sang to her or read her a story from the Disney Princess book that we bought her. I bought her things like that for every milestone, writing a message inside so that she would always have that to reflect upon. I began collecting the sweetest figurines and snow globes for her during this time called Westland Dreamsicles. (She still has them, although they are tucked away in our attic. Maybe her future children will enjoy them.)

Sometimes I would just have conversations with her and the Lord while she would stare at me for as long as she could bear. I prayed aloud every chance I got so she could hear what I was saying. She seemed comforted by my voice, and I felt joy when her tiny blue eyes met mine. Although I was still trying to barter with God on occasion, I had succumbed to the fact that I could not change His mind and that I had very little control over Abi's circumstance.

My message inside Abi's Disney princess book

Psalm 91

Whoever dwells in the shelter of the Most High
will rest in the shadow of the Almighty.
I will say of the Lord, "He is my refuge and my fortress,
my God, in whom I trust."
Surely he will save you
from the fowler's snare
and from the deadly pestilence.
He will cover you with his feathers,
and under his wings you will find refuge;
his faithfulness will be your shield and rampart.
You will not fear the terror of night,
nor the arrow that flies by day,
nor the pestilence that stalks in the darkness,
nor the plague that destroys at midday.
A thousand may fall at your side,
ten thousand at your right hand,
but it will not come near you.
You will only observe with your eyes
and see the punishment of the wicked.
If you say, "The Lord is my refuge,"
and you make the Most High your dwelling,
no harm will overtake you,
no disaster will come near your tent.
For he will command his angels concerning you
to guard you in all your ways;
they will lift you up in their hands,
so that you will not strike your foot against a stone.
You will tread on the lion and the cobra;
you will trample the great lion and the serpent.
"Because he loves me," says the Lord, "I will rescue him;
I will protect him, for he acknowledges my name.
He will call on me, and I will answer him;
I will be with him in trouble,

I will deliver him and honor him.
With long life I will satisfy him
and show him my salvation."

My favorite part of the Bible to read to Abi was Psalm 91. It meant so much to me that I had it tattooed on my left wrist. This prayer of protection gave me great comfort during this part of my life, and reinforced my faith that God was in total control, even in the worst circumstances.

With my breast pump dangling from my unharmed left shoulder, I would take frequent strolls to the nursing room, guided by my wheeled walker. There, I would pump all the milk that my battered body could produce and store it in my refrigerated bag until I could transport it to the shelf marked "Slater" in the Rainbow House freezer. I was never as shocked as the first time I opened that commercial-sized freezer, designed specifically for breast milk, and saw shelf after shelf of eight-ounce bottles filled to the brim with what we moms called "liquid gold." It was like a NICU baby's heaven!

Around lunch time, Brian and Noah would come to the hospital to eat lunch as a family in the cafeteria. Eating meals as a family was always important to me. The hospital gave me $5 coupons for every meal that I ate in the cafeteria as a reward for being a breastfeeding mother—a nice perk of which all the NICU moms took advantage.

Other Families in Our New Community

After lunch, Brian and Noah would go back to Rainbow House, where Noah would play with some of the other children staying there with their families. I specifically remember a little boy named Gabe, about four years old, who had leukemia. Fair-skinned, with no hair or eyebrows but the energy of a healthy young boy, Gabe brought a ray of light to every room he entered.

He was always such an energetic soul, with beams of light just bursting from every inch of his tender little body. He and his parents never stayed for more than a few days at a time—just long enough for Gabe to receive his treatments and rest a bit. Then they would be gone for a week or two before returning for more treatments. When Gabe and his family would leave to go back home, Noah would be lost. He talked about Gabe constantly until he came back for a visit, and then Noah would be on cloud nine again. Noah has no recollection of Gabe now, but at the time, they were inseparable. I wonder about him—did he beat his disease and grow up to attend college, like Noah did? I choose to believe he did.

When dinnertime approached, it was time for me to say good night to my baby girl, the nurses, and other NICU parents. I would peek in from time to time on some of the other babies and their families. Being in similar situations, it seemed inevitable that we would form bonds with one another. And because the NICU at Children's Hospital of Omaha was nothing more than one gigantic room with divider walls, we couldn't help but overhear conversations.

On one particular day— it was a gloomy, rainy day as I remember it—I happened to overhear the very young parents in the pod next to Abigail's as they experienced something every parent hopes never to bear. Their little one was born with all the odds stacked against him, mostly due to genetic impairments, as I recall. They made the decision to take their tiny baby off life support, and it was more than I could handle when they made the call to order the baby's casket. I will never forget that moment for as long as I live. My stomach felt sick while I tried to drown out their voices—I was heartbroken for them. The parents were teenagers and I heard someone, maybe one of their own parents, say to them, "You were too young to have a baby anyway." Oh my gosh, it broke me. I cried and called Brian to get a ride back to Rainbow House. I felt like an intruder in their most private, heart-wrenching experience. I needed to get out of there immediately and retreat to my safe place with my husband and son.

Brian and Noah picked me up, and we headed back to Rainbow House for dinner, just as we did most nights. Some nights, especially when we wanted to feel more like a normal family, we would eat dinner at the Applebee's just down the street from the hospital and Rainbow House. But on that particular night, I got my dinner from the kitchen in Rainbow House, and ate it in my room, completely alone.

I realized that when we are in a situation like the one Brian, Noah, and I experienced, although life may seem impossible in the present, we are blessed nonetheless. Things are never as bad as they seem, and they can always be worse. A person never has to look far to find someone in a worse situation. Not that it's necessarily a good thing, but it's all about perspective, right? Everyone can use a hug or a smile once in a while, and you should never let the opportunity slip by—you never know when or if it will come again. We just never know what others are experiencing, so we learn to always be kind.

As I reflected on what occurred on that day, I realized I had gained a new perspective in my own experience with my family and with my new baby girl's prognosis. As impossible as things seemed at times, we were blessed to still cling to hope for a future with Abi, while those young parents could not. It gave me a new appreciation for how fortunate we were and taught me that we never really know what others are experiencing in life. Compassion and kindness to all should always be at the core of our values, and I vowed to practice that in my daily life moving forward. To this day, I pray every morning and night in gratitude for everything I have been given.

The Caring Staff and Volunteers

Volunteers came to Rainbow House most nights and either cooked for the guests, or brought in carry-out meals at their expense. We never went hungry, thanks to the care of the volunteers; they provided everything we could have wanted and more. The Rainbow House staff and volunteers poured themselves into the needs of those who stayed there, listening to our woes when we needed a shoulder to cry on. They had seen so much that they were rarely shocked by anything we told them. Those men and women were truly unique people, and I often wonder if they had any idea how much of a beautiful difference they made in our otherwise chaotic and emotional worlds.

When I think about our experience during the first two months of Abigail's life, some of my fondest memories were of Rainbow House, its staff, and volunteers. I honestly do not know how we would have made it through Abi's hospital stay had it not been for the shelter and compassion of those wonderful people. I can remember thinking to myself during our stay there that if I were ever in a position to volunteer at a place like Rainbow House (I have since learned that these places are called Hospitality Houses), I would give back in the same manner that I experienced. In fact, as I write these words, I am now a member of the board of directors of the Family House in Peoria, Illinois, where I am able to do just that. Isn't life spectacular when you can see it come full circle?

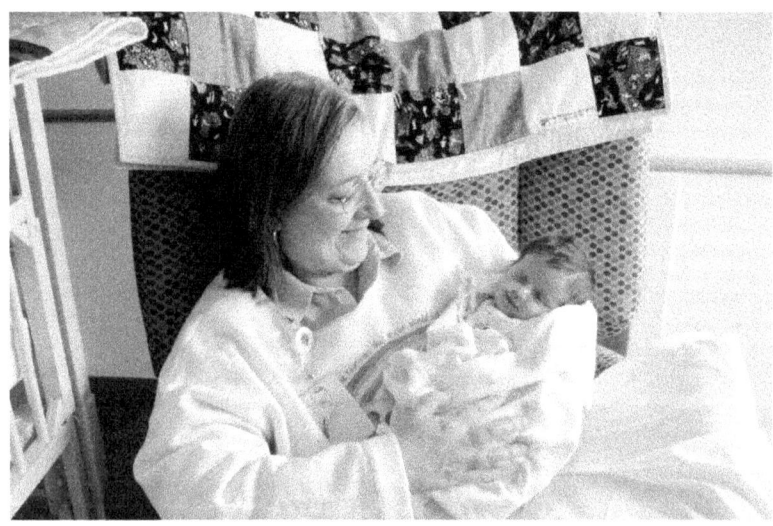

Abi with one of the sweet employees at Rainbow House

Noah's Discoveries

After dinner, Brian would take his shift in Abi's room, and Noah and I would lounge around Rainbow House. It overflowed with fun things to do, and we took advantage of it as often as we were able. We would play in the large playroom that joined the kitchen and dining areas. I could sit at a dining table with other parents while Noah played with kiddos who also had siblings in the hospital, never losing sight of him.

I liked to read books with Noah and spend quality time with him when I was not with Abi. I wanted him to feel safe and peaceful. I don't think he ever really understood what was happening. He just went along with whatever we did and never seemed to mind. At his young age, his world had changed suddenly and without warning. My hope was that he never felt confused or uncomfortable. It was several weeks before he really seemed to understand that he had a new baby sister who lived in the hospital. The day he was finally able to meet her for the first time was the same day that she had her first shunt surgery, November 14, 2002, and Abigail was nearly one month old. To protect her from exposure to new germs outside of the NICU, the nurses wheeled her down the hallway to the OR in an Isolette. Accompanied by Brian and me, Noah peered at her through the glass, said a quick "Hi, Abi," and then off she went.

As for me, I was dealing with something totally foreign too. My independence had been stolen from me, and I was subjected to feeling like an invalid to everyone, at least that's how I saw it. Brian was solid throughout the whole experience and never complained about having to care for two dependent people, but 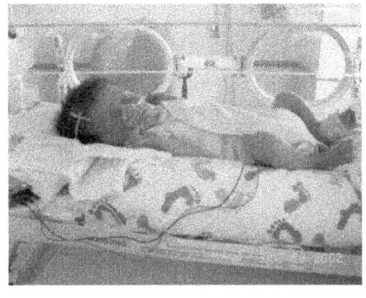 Noah could not understand why I wasn't able to hold him when he wanted to be held or carried when he was tired of walking. He wondered what the walker and wheelchair were for and thought it was funny when Brian pushed me in the chair over long distances.

On Halloween night, we took Noah to the "Boo at the Zoo" event in Omaha, where he wore his Buzz Lightyear costume, collected candy, and played games with other children his age. Since the night involved much more walking than I could participate in with my wheeled companion, Brian swiped a wheelchair from the hospital and pushed me alongside Noah as he had his Halloween fun. He became tired, and since I had a fresh dose of pain meds, I allowed him to sit on my lap as Brian pushed us along. Noah thought this was great fun and did not want to give up the fun ride in the strange-looking chair on wheels.

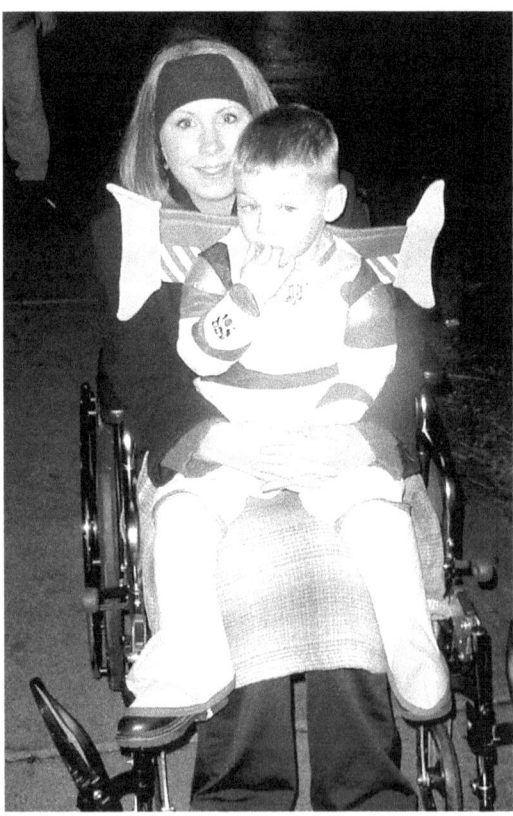

Noah and me at Boo at the Zoo

The Invalid Mother

Bedtime was always the worst part of the day for me because I never slept well and often woke during the night after horrible dreams. I saw that red semi every time I closed my eyes, but swore to myself and everyone around me that I did not need anti-anxiety drugs or a therapist to get me through this. (After 11 months, I gave that idea up and took advantage of both.) I wept a multitude of tears, mostly at night, for the physical and mental anguish that I was experiencing. When my mom would stay with us, I would often wake up sobbing when my pain medication was wearing off, and she would lovingly help me take more of the correct type and number of pills. I loved having my own personal nurse around when Mom could afford the time off work to make the trip. And I know she loved taking care of me as that's what she felt she was born to do: take care of others.

For about six weeks after the accident, I had to sleep in a fortress of pillows at night. My mother was there to move them when needed. If I moved at all without the pillows there to stabilize me, it felt as if my bones were collapsing beneath me. I will always remember the sound the bones would make when the pillows weren't where they needed to be—they crackled and crunched in the most obnoxious way.

When I woke during the night to use the bathroom, Brian or my mom would have to assist me to be sure that I didn't fall or accidentally pee on myself because I was unable to get out of bed independently. How humiliating!

My walker was always parked beside the bed, and I would get to a point where I would give it all I had to get out of bed on my own but I would usually end up defeated. I cried every time I had to move, especially to get out of bed. It was such a chore that I joked about wearing adult diapers so that I would only have to deal with the pain in the morning. Inevitably, I would be up several times throughout the night and despised the idea of waking someone for help, though I had no choice.

When independence is taken from someone who has always been driven from within, it can be the worst type of torture.

Morning always came much too soon, leaving me exhausted yet motivated by the very thought of seeing my frail baby daughter. The sheer task of getting myself prepared in the mornings was treacherous and tedious. It took me so long to get from point A to point B within the room that I had to be sure to choose Noah's and my clothing the night before to save 15 minutes the next morning. Unable to shower myself in the beginning, either Brian or Mom was right beside me. I had become dependent on Brian for nearly everything. He would shave my legs, bathe me, and even wash my hair for the first few weeks. Because of my rotator cuff injury, raising my right arm was not an option until it was rehabilitated in physical therapy. To this day, I have problems with my right shoulder and wrist if I do not do exercises to keep them strong, and I have worsening arthritis in my hips.

After I was a bit more independent, I would walk myself into the bathroom and sit down on the bench in the shower to bathe myself. Though seemingly insignificant to others, this was an incredible win for me. Still, it would take a considerable amount of time just to shower myself; I would spend the better part of 25 minutes showering if I did it independently. Getting dressed on my own was something that would come along later. I needed assistance, especially putting my pants on and getting my top over my head. My morning routine normally took an hour and a half, provided I had all the prep work done the prior night. Again, many things are taken for granted when you are not physically impaired. I am thankful that my impairment was only temporary, and I never take for granted the ability to use my body now that I know what being impaired feels like.

My First Solo Exploration

With this newfound independence came a strong will not to burden my husband any more than I already had. I will always vividly remember one bitterly cold, dark, snowy morning after

Mom had returned to Illinois. Brian was sleeping so soundly that the thought of waking him to chauffeur me to the place that held my daughter hostage made me do the unthinkable: I got myself ready and walked to the hospital. Exhausted and feeling as though I had been hit by a freight train (oh, wait—I guess I *had* been hit by a couple of semitrucks!), I clumsily pulled myself out of bed, immediately taking every pain med that was allowed. My clothes were just as I had laid them the night before and I flung them over the handle of my walker, making my way into the bathroom where I triumphantly got myself dressed and ready for the day.

Since neither Brian nor Noah stirred during my morning ritual, I decided I would walk the half mile from Rainbow House to the Children's Hospital, accompanied only by my winter coat and walker. This would be the first time—but not the last—that I would pretend to be the superhero that I absolutely was not, and for that, I would later pay dearly. Cold and growing increasingly tired and winded with each laborious step, I made my way through the snow to my baby. My salty tears froze on my face just as soon as they left my eyes and the wind stung my skin, but I knew I could not turn back. Desperate to regain some level of independence, I kept trudging through the snow, as badly as my body rebelled against me. This had to be the dumbest thing I could have done, but it meant momentarily experiencing my evasive independence.

When I finally arrived at the fourth floor of the hospital, I must have appeared even more awful than I felt because the nursing staff rushed to my side to assist me in my trek to Abigail's side. They threw daggers at me with their eyes, asking questions like, "What in the world were you thinking?" when I told them what I had done. I didn't care. I was now where I needed to be and that was all that mattered to me, although my poor body was approaching a state of shock and frostbite. I knew I would be in trouble once Brian awoke to find that I was gone, but I could deal with that when that time came. For now, I would enjoy the fruits of my labor in the way I had many mornings before sitting next to my daughter's bed with my Bible and my prayers.

Parenting 2.0

The nursing staff had to teach Brian and me how to handle our fragile little girl, which was different from handling a typical newborn. For example, we were taught how to hold Abigail correctly because of all the cords and monitors that had become an integral part of her existence. The nurses taught us a certain technique to bathe her as well, given her physical state. Because she was tiny with a compromised immune system, she could easily catch a cold, so we bathed her wrapped in a towel inside a miniature tub of warm water. She loved those warm baths, and we loved being able to touch her and bond in a way we hadn't before.

Leading up to the bottle, Abi only received feedings intravenously and then via feeding tube. After she graduated from the feeding tube to bottles, we learned to feed her correctly. Her first bottles were miniature and when she first began drinking, she would only take a couple of drops. While we were able to celebrate a few things, there was still a long distance to travel at this stage of her life.

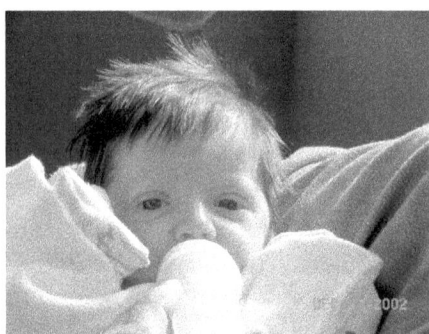 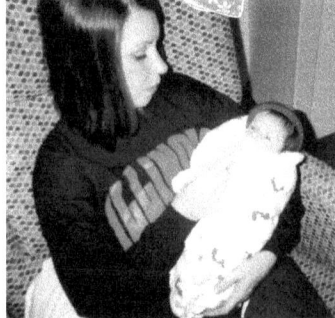

The Shunt

Abigail's neurosurgeon "pulled up a chair" in November, indicating that we were about to have a serious discussion. He explained to us that the inevitable was upon us since her ventricles were still becoming increasingly enlarged and her head circumference was growing with no end in sight. The neurosurgery team decided it was time to place the shunt, a concept to which we had been introduced only weeks before. A tube designed to assist her body in draining the cerebrospinal fluid from her head to her abdomen would be inserted in her head, allowing the excess fluid to be excreted with her waste. To do this, they not only had to perform brain surgery to place the shunt in the ventricle, but they also had to make two incisions to insert the tube that would carry the fluid downward—one incision was in her neck and the other in her abdomen.

The surgery would occur on November 14, 2002, at 1:00 p.m. That meant I had a few days to plead with God to take this all away, removing the need for surgery. I thought that if I begged long enough and hard enough, He would perform a miracle right before our eyes and make all the fluid drain on its own. God doesn't normally work that way, no matter how much begging and pleading we do. He will always do things His way and in His own perfect time. Nonetheless, I would give it all I had, hoping for a miracle and claiming victory as if it were already in the works. It couldn't hurt, right?

Well, November 14 came and there was no sign of the miracle for which I had been desperately praying. The surgery took place, and Abigail became the new proud owner of her very first programmable ventriculoperitoneal (VP) shunt—just what every girl dreams of! It was placed on the left side of her head, just above her ear, and from the moment she first received it, it was nothing but trouble. We noticed that fluid was slowly seeping from her fresh head wounds, but we assumed that all would be well. The neurosurgeons that made their rounds would inspect it and see that the fluid continued to seep into her hair.

They would apply an exterior sort of gel, much like super glue, in hopes that it would remedy the issue. This was something we continued to watch.

While Abi recovered from her first shunt surgery, we had the privilege of celebrating Thanksgiving with our friends at Rainbow House, and Dad traveled to be with us too since we always spent the holiday with our families in Illinois. Mom stayed behind to be with my brothers for the holiday. Again, the staff and volunteers put great effort into providing a beautiful experience for those of us who called Rainbow House our home away from home. They prepared more food than we could all consume in one day: multiple turkeys with all the traditional fixings like green bean casserole, sweet potatoes, stuffing, pies—what a spread! It smelled like Thanksgiving, and it looked like Thanksgiving, but it just wasn't the same as we had grown accustomed to. It was only one holiday, though, right?

Visitors, Kind Words, and Beautiful Gestures

Throughout our stay in Omaha, we were blessed by the company of a few visitors from Illinois. My dad made the six-and-a-half-hour trek alone on most weekends, and I cherished the time he spent with Abi and me in her NICU room. We would begin our mornings on those weekends with a trip to Starbucks in the mall just down the street from the hospital and settle in for hours of R & R with our silent little companion.

Throughout my childhood, the relationship that I had with my dad served as the foundation upon which I built my relationships with other men in my life. He was someone I adored and looked up to for as long as I could remember, and the way he treated my mother showed me what I wanted in a spouse. When Mom and us kids needed anything at all, Dad always made sure we were well cared for. It was inspiring to see that my daughter already had the same type of relationship with him, and I enjoyed watching him interact with her in a way that only he could. What amazed me the most was the fact that it came so naturally for him. There was never a question whether or not he would be there, and I knew that being with us meant just as much to him as it did to me. Anyone who knew my dad knew that one of his many gifts was keeping the mood light. While there were many times that I wanted to wallow in self-pity like a pig rolls in mud, he would never allow it. My mom, brothers, and I always came first in Dad's life, and we never wondered how much he loved us. He was my real-life Superman (until Brian came along, that is).

My mom came as often as she could, too. As a nurse, she always had a natural desire and ability to take care of people, and that is exactly what she did for me and my family. She traveled by train all the way from Monmouth to help out however she could when Dad couldn't accompany her. Driving alone on a highway for that long distance was not something she felt comfortable doing, but it didn't stop her from coming to see us. She would serve as Noah's caregiver, our housekeeper, and then would sneak away to visit Abi when all of the business was taken care of. I knew that it was difficult for her to see us in such a dire situation, which gave me an even greater appreciation for her selfless efforts. I hope she knew how loved and valued she was by my little family and me. She was a force!

Other visitors from Illinois included Brian's dad and his dad's wife, and my cousin Chrissy. My brother Nathan visited once we were back home from the hospital when Abi was more stable. A few local friends and coworkers would occasionally stop by to check in on us and see if we needed anything. Often, they would bring gifts, never forgetting about Noah when they arrived with clothes or stuffed animals for Abi. Their visits made a world of difference for us all. Since most of them lived in or around Lincoln, it was unbelievable to me that they cared enough to take the time to visit us in Omaha. Although we had only been residents of Nebraska for a short time, we had made amazing friends who would remain so for a very long time.

We received countless cards from loved ones at home as the

news of our accident spread, as well as from those local to our new community. Our church family in Illinois sent notes filled with prayers for Abi's and my recovery, which were read daily, and my hospital room was abundantly decorated with incredibly vibrant floral arrangements. The love and concern showered upon us from many parts of the country was overwhelming and added joy to my otherwise gloomy disposition. I felt blessed then, and I remain in awe of the generosity that we experienced.

Discharge

Abigail remained a resident of the Children's Hospital NICU, Room 470 until December 1, 2002. After three blood transfusions, placement of a central line, and placement of a VP shunt, evaluation for possible Hirschsprung's disease (a condition in the large intestine that causes difficulty passing waste), and countless tests and procedures for various other medical conditions, we were given the consent to leave the premises with our nearly two-month-old baby girl. We were heading home.

I was cautiously optimistic to be leaving the hospital, but still felt some hesitation when my dad and I packed up my perfectly flawed infant while Brian was working. Following the transportation instructions of the hospital nursing staff, I strapped the now five-pound bundle of joy into her infant carrier and fastened her brother into his car seat for the ride. Anxiously, the four of us made the trek from Omaha back to Lincoln in hopes of finding some sense of normalcy in our quaint duplex, which eagerly awaited our return.

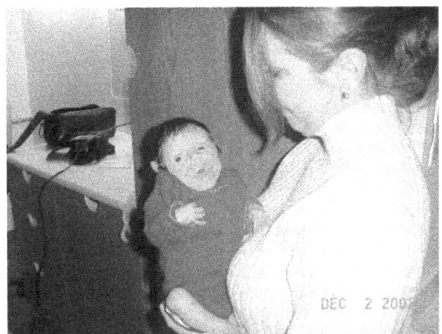 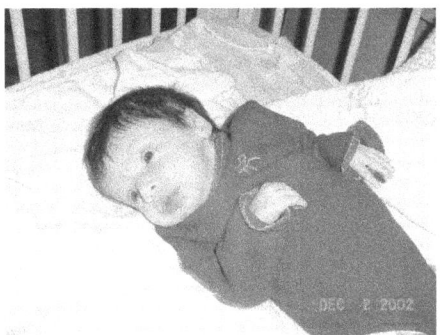

Abi and me on our last day in the NICU

To learn more about the medical terms and
topics discussed in this chapter, visit this link:

www.SavingAbigailGrace.com

CHAPTER FIVE

Back Home... Or So We Thought

ENTERING OUR HOME THAT DREARY December morning, with my mechanically-augmented baby in tow, was another bittersweet moment for me. While I was excited to move on to the newest chapter of our lives at home as a family, I was filled to the brim with anxiety and worry—anxiety about what was next now that I would not have a full medical staff to rely on at all hours of the day and night; worry that something would go wrong and we would have to return to Rainbow House. Call it mother's intuition.

The cold air inside the duplex stung our faces as if we were standing outside. To save money on utility bills, Brian had shut the furnace down while we were living in Omaha, and neither of us had had a chance to prepare the place for a more welcoming return. A home that would typically smell of dinner cooking, holiday candles burning, and cookies baking now reeked of stale air and decaying plant matter. All the flowers that friends and family had sent me while I stayed at Bryan LGH—once beautiful and vibrant, now dead—covered the dining room table. The spiritual parallel of the moment was not lost on me. My surroundings mirrored exactly what I felt inside: my broken-down, damaged family, the cold ambient air, and the smell of rotted, lifeless flowers surrounded my weary soul. But no matter how anxious and tired I felt in that moment, I knew my top priority would be getting my tiny princess settled right away.

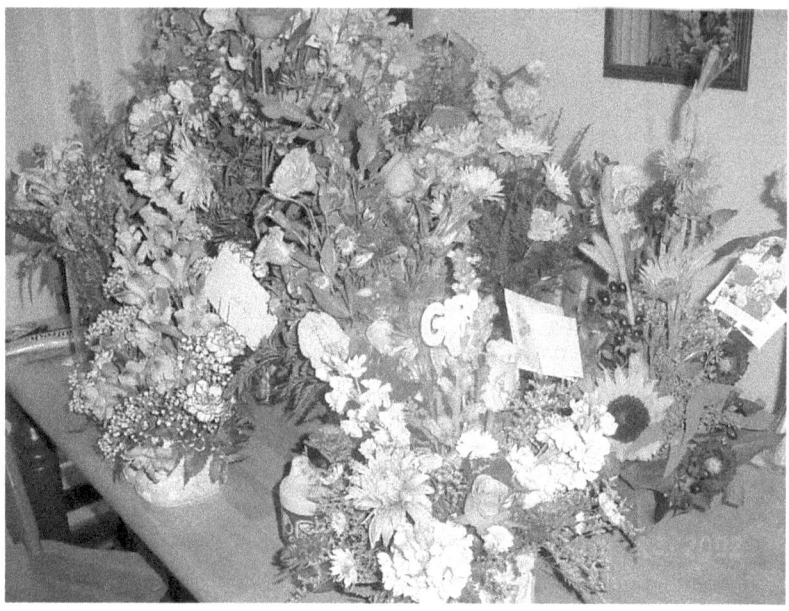

As my dad, Noah, and I dropped our bags inside the front door, I was a ball of nerves, apprehensively reflecting upon all of the discharge instructions that accompanied this tiny person, whom, until today, I had only been allowed to touch in the presence of medical personnel. My stomach was in knots, and I couldn't shake the intense feeling of dread that was churning in my belly. Knowing that I had much to do and little energy with which to do it—and with Dad leaving soon—I had no choice but to dig deep for strength. The house hadn't been cleaned in a month and a half. The dining table would need to be cleared off for dinner, which would also need to be prepared soon. My toddler son had pent-up energy to burn, and my fussy baby girl needed the warmth of her mama, a comfort which she had been deprived of for too long. Cleaning could wait, and come to think of it, so could dinner.

Before being discharged from the hospital, Abi was in a relatively stable state, especially considering her entrance into this world was not meant to be for yet another four days. The notes sent home by the medical staff read that her *heart rate is regular and without murmur*, her *suture sites are healing well*, her *chest is clear*, her *tone is adequate*, and her color is normal, *though the patient seems slightly weak*. Her abdomen was still distended (enlarged), and what was originally referred to as possible Hirschsprung's disease had been dismissed, although she was still not having regular bowel movements. The only diagnosis to come of this irregularity was a small bowel obstruction. The doctors reported no further leakage of fluid at the incision sites where her shunt had been placed, but the small wet spot under her head on the car seat pillow indicated otherwise.

Abi was given a brand-new bag of blood immediately preceding her release, as well as a fresh shot of Synagis (palivizumab—a precautionary drug given to most preemies to arm them against RSV, or respiratory syncytial virus, a potentially fatal infant illness) in the hope that her health would improve as she adapted to life outside the hospital. She would need additional intramuscular doses monthly for the next five months to sufficiently protect her from becoming critically ill.

The notes from the doctors were good news, but I had some major concerns. *Is it my imagination, or does she look jaundiced? Maybe she is just overwhelmed, but does she seem a bit lethargic? My senses are probably just overactive, but if the shunt site is supposed to be healed, why is there still some oozing in her fine, dark hair?* Until now, she had only rarely been free from the cords and wires connected to huge machines, buzzing from the work they did throughout each day and night. *How will she do without them?*

Up to this point, I had been able to rely on the guidance of one specialist after another, knowing they were always there if something went wrong. And while I was elated that Abi's medical team was comfortable releasing us to our new doctors "on the outside," I was nervous. *How will I manage without them?* Now,

I only had my own knowledge and skills to rely on for most of the day. This terrified me to the core.

By now, Brian was back to his regular work schedule, hitting the ground running and plugging away from 6:00 a.m. until 6:30 p.m., sometimes even later. His job had been in jeopardy because of all the time he had missed while Abigail and I were recovering in the hospitals. As branch manager of a large fleet of rental cars with multiple employees, he was needed to keep things operating smoothly. And back then, there was no such thing as paternity leave, at least not as we know it today, even though the Family and Medical Leave Act (FMLA) was nearly 10 years old at that time. Even if Brian could have taken time off without risking his career, he would still need a paycheck, as our medical bills were piling up more every day.

An Unexpected Blessing

Thankfully, the federal agency I worked for (NRCS) had an amazing program that allowed employees in situations similar to mine to use a bank where other employees could transfer their unused paid time off (PTO). After being informed of our situation through the human resources office, our story struck a chord with many of my coworkers nationally, and they were happy to help. The sympathy and goodwill of the NRCS employees was nothing short of a miracle in itself.

My human resources department worked everything out for me, and each day there would be more time banked in my portal because of the kindness of people across the United States that had never even met me. As a result of their incredible generosity, after exhausting all my own PTO, I was still able to get full paychecks for nearly four months. This gave me the chance to focus on my and Abi's healing at home, without the added stress of returning to work before I was ready or worrying about losing my job.

To put that into perspective, my NRCS coworkers had decidedly parted with approximately 680 hours of PTO to make sure my family and I were financially cared for. The kindness of those strangers will forever be etched in my memory and in my heart. I am grateful for the NRCS employees who made our trauma tolerable in such a beautiful way.

Keeping My Kiddos Safe

I had new doctors and specialists to introduce to Abigail: a new pediatrician, a pediatric neurosurgeon for follow-up appointments, and a pediatric ophthalmologist. I also had my own appointments to make with my orthopedic specialist and physical therapist. All these appointments were made so they did not expose my RSV-susceptible infant to the elements. (It was December in Nebraska, where there was always a likelihood of snow and ice, as well as people with cold and flu symptoms.) I had to keep her indoors, away from human contact, since her immune system was still very fragile and even the smallest bug could prove fatal to her. It would have eased my anxiety if medical personnel could visit our home, sparing us the of risk of illness every time we left our sterile surroundings.

I have no doubt that this was about the time that I developed a self-diagnosed case of obsessive-compulsive disorder (OCD). The thought of germs living in my home and causing harm to my sweet little girl turned me into a cleaning Tasmanian devil. It was more than keeping up with toys that were out of place or dirty dishes; I was armed with bleach and Lysol all day, every day. I bleached the countertops in the kitchen every time Brian or I used them. I wiped down every surface with antibacterial wipes and sprayed doorknobs and faucets with Lysol in every room as soon as they were touched by human hands. I must have washed my hands hundreds of times throughout those days.

To make matters worse, my little boy did not understand why his toys got daily antibacterial baths. Noah longed for a normal life and routine, hoping we would pick up where we left off almost two months ago. Honestly, we all needed that. Thankfully, God blessed us with the sweetest little boy who was easily entertained by his Hot Wheels and Matchbox cars. In fact, there was never a moment when he was not carrying one in his hand. He was content to be home in the company of his mommy, daddy, and now his baby sister. He would also prove to be a handy little assistant to his mommy and sister in the days ahead. His love for Abigail and his concern for her well-being would always be unmatched.

Dad Leaves and My Intuition Is Validated

After my two little ones and I were safely home from the hospital, it was time for my dad to make the seven-and-a-half-hour drive from Lincoln to his home in Illinois, where my mom was eagerly awaiting his arrival. My stomach was in knots and the air felt heavy, like the weight of the world was pushing down on my body. Having my dad around always gave me the most intense feeling of safety and security, and his undying light-heartedness made even the weariest soul feel comforted. He didn't need to say a word; there was just something craveable about his presence. Of course, my dad would have been a great help if he had been able to stay longer, but he needed to return to his job.

Before he left, we hugged for a moment (Dad was never big on physical affection), and I cried hot tears onto his shoulder. He laughed it off and said, "I'll be back soon. You're gonna be fine."

I could hardly bear to watch Dad walk out the door, and I knew that it was probably harder for him to leave me in that moment. He hated being far away from me and my family; he loved us all deeply. I will never forget the moment after he closed the front door behind him. For the first time since my accident, I found myself utterly alone. I wept uncontrollably while my baby girl slept, and my toddler played with his cars beside me. I remember praying to God for the strength to pull our lives back together because it felt like everyone was relying on me for stability. Brian had to focus on his job to make ends meet financially, and I knew it would be up to me to piece everything together, at least for now.

That night, after Dad left and Brian returned from work, we got the "four-of-us-at-home" moment that we had desired for so long. Our family was together in our own house for the first time since the accident, and it felt surreal. By the grace of God, I had somehow managed to get some cleaning done and freshened the stale air, replacing it with the smell of dinner (and bleach). We sat around the table that, just hours earlier, had served as a flower cemetery, and reveled in the color that was brought back into the dining room by the veggies that donned our plates. Picture this: a home-cooked meal with my husband, son, and new daughter—all of us finally together after 45 nights of eating at the Rainbow House table, Applebee's, or in the hospital cafeteria. Noah sat in his highchair without a care in his beautiful head, while Abi sat propped up in her car seat between my and Brian's chairs, enabling her to be part of this momentous occasion. It was almost like our own living version of a Norman Rockwell painting.

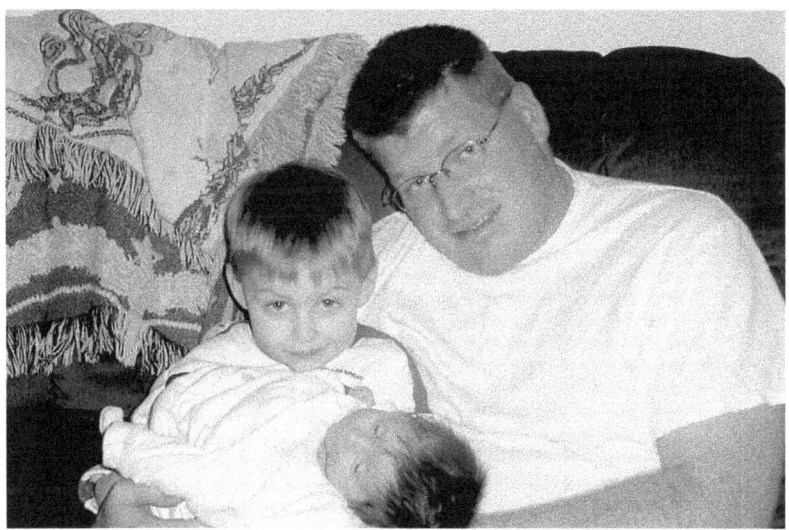

Our first night home

We had missed putting the Christmas tree up that day— something we always did on December 1—and would do it the next day instead. It would be Abi's first Christmas, which was very exciting. Brian and I cleaned up our dinner mess, I bleached the kitchen again, and we loved on our little family in the small living room next to a cozy fire. Life felt lovely in that moment, and I ate it up like it was birthday cake with ice cream. The heavy air that lingered in the duplex after Dad left was suddenly clean and light and filled with the scent of hope and contentment. I didn't want it to end.

After being home for less than 24 hours, however, my ear-

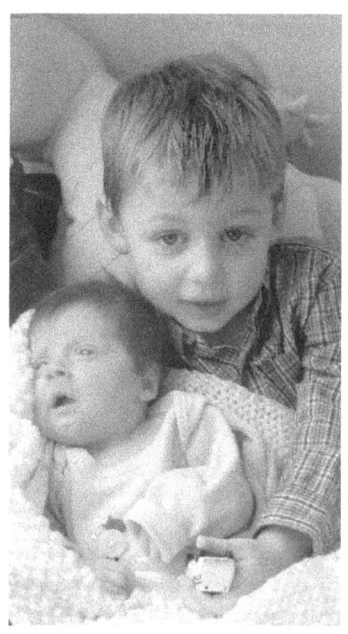

Noah holding his very sick sister

lier intuition proved valid. Abigail looked sickly: her skin was discolored and she was lethargic. Her belly looked extremely bloated, and I could see in her eyes that she was incredibly uncomfortable. She was running a high fever and seemed almost lifeless. By December 3, two days after our release from the Children's Hospital, we were in the emergency room with concerns that her shunt was malfunctioning or infected. I was terrified of losing this precious gift God had entrusted to me. I feared I was on the verge of failing my child once again.

I believe that everything happens for a reason and knew there had to be one for not finding the time to put up the Christmas tree. There would be no holiday smells or Christmas lights in our home this year. God had other plans for our holiday season, and they did not include baking cookies together to share with the neighbors, as had always been our tradition. Nor did they include gathering in our home or the homes of friends and family for fellowship and reflection over tasty dishes like the green bean casserole and sweet potato casserole my mom always made. Nope, not this year! When your baby girl is as sick as mine was, those plans evade your reality like smoke escaping from a fire.

Back in the PICU

After a long stay in the emergency room that night, Abigail was admitted to the Children's Hospital again for the medical staff to run tests and analyze blood work to determine the cause of her illness. After enduring yet another round of needles, poking, prodding, wires, cords, and machines, there was no conclusive evidence of any major health concerns, and we were sent on our merry way once again with instructions to call if her health worsened. We were told to look for signs of a shunt infection or malfunction which included high fever, vomiting, and what they called "sundown eyes," because the eyes appear to be looking downward. If I thought I was nervous coming home from the hospital the first time, the feeling was now intensified. I was absolutely beside myself with worry and had such an unsettling feeling in my gut that we would be back again soon.

After being in the NICU for 45 days, and then moving to the Pediatric Intensive Care Unit (PICU) from December 3 to 4, I was less than confident that this would be the end of Abigail's turbulent nightmare with hospital visits. Given her physical state, I had a feeling we would soon find ourselves back at Children's Hospital—and I was spot-on. While the rest of the country seemed to be thinking about the holiday season and all the joy it brings, we were preparing ourselves for the worst.

The day after being released, Abi's health once again deteriorated. Her temperature was 102.8 degrees, the discoloration of her skin had not improved, and her abdomen was tender and distended since she was still unable to excrete waste regularly. Two days after being sent home for the second time, we were making yet another journey from Lincoln to Omaha, and this time it was serious. We would again become residents of

Rainbow House and Abigail would be admitted to the PICU, this time for an extended stay.

As you can imagine, I relied heavily on the advice and guidance of our medical experts. Even when I had a gut feeling that something was "off" with my baby daughter, I tried to trust that all would be well. Sometimes I convinced myself that I was just overreacting to these "gut feelings" or what I thought was intuition.

Advocating For Your Child

Parents! I encourage you to trust your intuition and to always speak to your child's medical team if you feel that something is off with their health. As mothers, we have a bond with our babies like no other human could have because we carried them in our bodies. We become familiar with their movements as we feel them and watch them moving in our bellies. Even their personalities become somewhat familiar to us while they are growing inside their cocoons. We know if they will have laid-back personalities or if they will be busy once they are in the outside world. By the time we hold our babies in our arms for the first time, we already know them profoundly. Fathers also have a special bond with their children and your voice is valuable in their care.

Who better to advocate for them in this crazy, beautiful life than their parents? If you feel that a provider is not hearing you or that they are not taking your concerns seriously, speak up and make yourself understood. It may be difficult at times to articulate your rationale behind a feeling that you have, so finding the medical professionals that are willing to give credibility to those feelings is important.

There are also advocates that can help you to articulate the needs of your child more clearly and those resources are provided for you at the end of this chapter. Many hospitals have these professionals in the child life or social work departments, and others can be found in local nonprofit organizations. Look for them before you have a reason to: preparation is the key to a successful journey, especially in terms of your child's health.

Abi did have an infection in her shunt, found by analyzing her cerebrospinal fluid after tapping the shunt with a needle. The procedure she would endure to eradicate the infection was quite possibly the worst of them all. On December 6, the shunt was removed via a second brain surgery on a still-fragile infant who would have only been one day old had the pregnancy gone full term. An external shunt was placed on the top left side of her head, enabling her body to excrete the fluid from her brain.

The external shunt drained the cerebrospinal fluid from Abi's ventricles by way of an external tube that resembled a drinking straw. For the shunt to function properly, Abi's head, and consequently her shunt, was elevated above the container that housed the drainage from her brain. If, at any point during her stay, the shunt fell below the container, basic physics says the fluid would flow back down the tube and end up right where it started: Abi's ventricle. Imagine having to keep any patient in that position for her hospital stay—which ended up totaling 20 days!—let alone an infant. It was exhausting!

Over the next fourteen days, we would play yet another waiting game while Abi was intravenously pumped full of maximum-strength antibiotics to annihilate the bacteria present in her body. After the infection was gone, the pediatric neurology team placed a new shunt, this time on the right side of her brain.

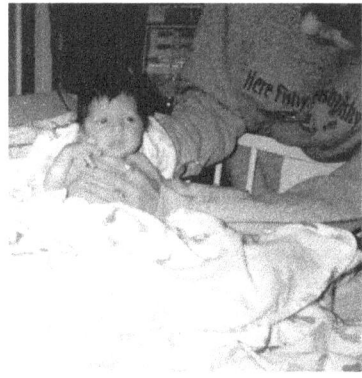
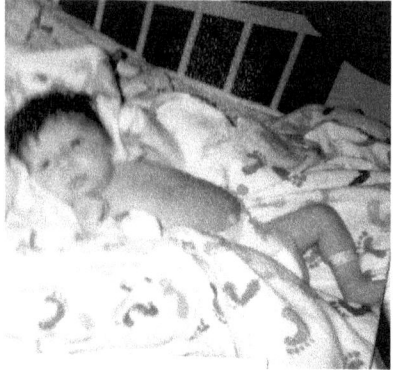
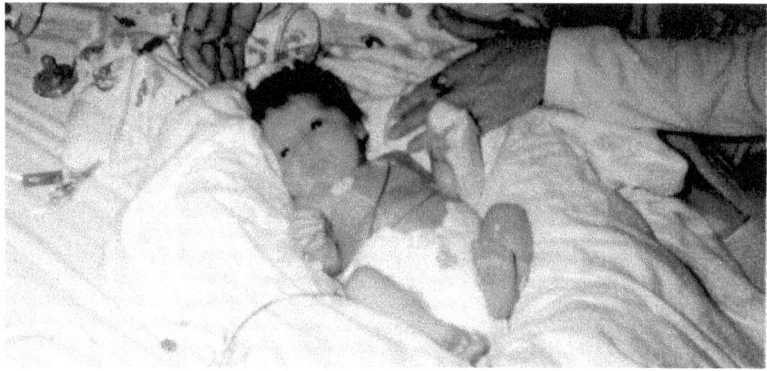

Shunt #2

In the meantime, my parents made the trip back to Omaha to support us, once again becoming invaluable to our otherwise gloomy existence. Every day, Abi was not only visited by the assigned nursing and doctoral staff, but was also entertained by the infectious disease and pediatric neurology teams. They performed daily tests on the fluid that had collected in the storage container, tracking the bacteria levels to see if they were decreasing.

While we waited for the infection to make its exit, Noah and I passed the time with toys, movies, and games that Children's Hospital provided for our entertainment. Brian visited when he could, but my poor husband was running on an empty tank all the time.

Somehow, despite his fatigue, he was always great at

making us laugh and keeping the mood light while we watched one day fade into the next.

Brian was managing the branch in Lincoln while we were in Omaha, driving daily between the two cities again. There were nights that I told him not to make the nearly 60-mile drive, for fear that he might fall asleep at the wheel. Still, there was nothing that could keep him away from the three of us, especially during the holidays. Christmastime had always been my husband's favorite time of the year, and that year was to be no different.

On December 20, 2002, Abigail became the recipient of her second VP shunt. She was observed continuously over the course of the next few days for fever, nausea, neurological issues, recurrence of infection, and other complications. While she was kept for observation, they also continued intravenous antibiotics as a precaution. If all went well and her body adjusted to the foreign system, we hoped to be home by Christmas. We prayed to be able to celebrate in our own traditional way, sans the Christmas tree and holiday decorations.

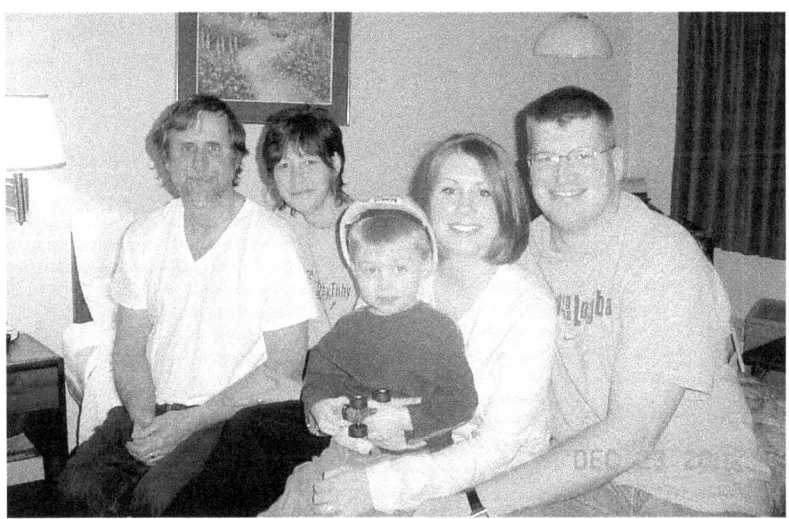

Christmas in Mom and Dad's hotel room

Christmas in the Rainbow House

As luck, or God's plan, would have it, we ended up spending yet another holiday in Omaha, away from our home. With my parents in town, we managed to spend our favorite holiday of the year together, even though we were all confined to their run-down hotel room just down the street from the hospital. My parents did not have a lot of money, but what they did have—and were more than happy to give us—was a great sense of humor and unending love and support. We exchanged gifts and managed to have a few laughs while our newest addition spent her first Christmas in a hospital bed with new mechanics in her brain.

The Rainbow House staff and volunteers made Christmas 2002 tolerable for those of us who were away from our homes and our own traditions by going all out to make us feel the spirit of the holiday. The house was decked out in decorations and the grand entry room featured a huge Christmas tree with loads of gifts underneath it—at least one for every man, woman, and child staying there. It even smelled like a traditional Christmas, with a feast of turkey and all the fixings prepared by folks who could have chosen to celebrate with their own families instead. With hearts of gold, they fed us, gave us gifts, and entertained us with songs, helping us forget, if only for one night, what was going on in our children's hospital rooms.

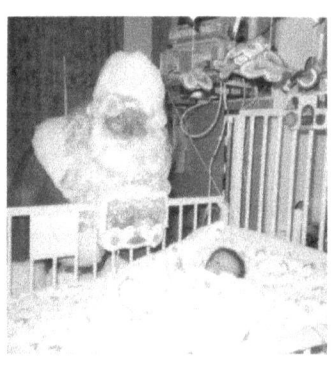

Although Abi wasn't allowed to spend her first Christmas with us at Rainbow House, she was visited by a precious volunteer dressed as Santa Claus, who handed out gifts to the children. He even had a gift for Noah, which brightened his day like nothing else could. Christmas was such a magical time of year, and my sweet boy was stuck away from home, so the mere sight of Santa that day put joy into his big blue eyes. Although I cannot remember the toy he received, I will forever remember the way it made my little boy's face gleam. What a blessing!

Mom and Dad stayed only a short while this time but whittled away many of the hours at Abi's bedside. It was much different in a PICU room than it was in the NICU. We were able to carefully hold her and play with her, being mindful of the vast number of new wounds that her tiny body displayed. She had a laceration on the left side of her head that she would wear proudly forever as a reminder of her failed shunt, as well as two sets of gashes on her neck and belly where the old and new shunt tubing were placed. Additionally, she wore newly sutured incisions where the most recent shunt was placed on the right side of her head just behind her ear.

Underneath the thin skin of her head, the mechanical part of the shunt system mimicked the shape of a matchbox car, which we found funny as we related it to Noah's addiction. But once her thick hair grew back, she would be the only one who could identify its whereabouts, which would become increasingly important as she aged.

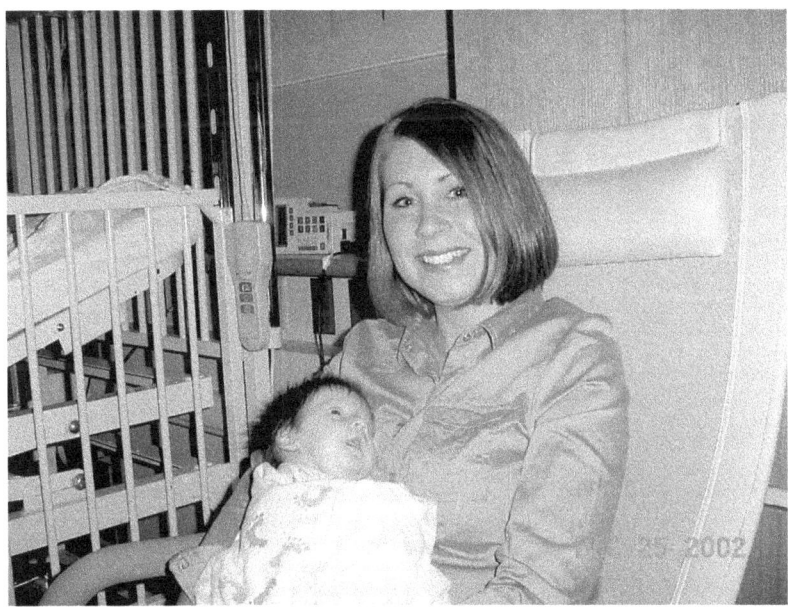

On December 26, 2002, the moment we had all anticipated with overwhelming emotions was upon us; Abigail was released from Children's Hospital. After packing our things and cleaning our room at Rainbow House, we were on our way back to a place we used to call home in Lincoln. Of course, we were sent home with more instructions on how to care for our little miracle baby upon discharge. We needed to follow up in two to three weeks with a cranial ultrasound and watch for any signs that her body was rejecting its new plastic work of art, like fever, chills, or wound drainage. Piece of cake, right? Add that to the already overwhelming task of bringing home a six-and-a-half-pound preemie with one incredibly complex medical history, and it was downright terrifying. But, shaking in my boots, we were homeward bound, and I was eager to move into the next chapter of our ever-evolving lives.

To learn more about the medical terms and topics discussed in this chapter, visit this link:

www.SavingAbigailGrace.com

CHAPTER SIX

A New "Normal"

BACK AT HOME, ANXIETY OVERWHELMED me as I faced the enormous responsibility of caring not only for myself—still healing from my own injuries—but also for my fragile newborn and toddler son. Brian was needed at work now more than ever, and his hours away from home would leave much to be desired by all members of our delicate family. It had now been more than two months since the accident occurred, and with Brian missing a significant amount of work in his role as branch manager, the branch suffered financially. When I was admitted to the hospital immediately following the accident, Brian's regional manager had assured him in the heat of the moment that she would take care of his branch and keep him informed of its happenings. Upon his return, he found that no such thing had occurred. The fleet of cars had decreased, and his employees were managed like cats being herded by a monkey. The pressure on Brian was more intense than ever. He was expected to turn things around in a very short amount of time, and if he could not, he would face severe consequences.

My employer, on the other hand, could not have handled the situation any better. While I was recovering in the hospital and nursing my baby daughter back to health, my HR representative worked tirelessly to make sure regular paychecks were deposited into my checking account. To Brian and me, the money was a gift from God. Without the income my employer provided, we could have easily lost our duplex rental. Our landlords weren't particularly empathetic toward our situation or the fact that we hadn't lived in our home for two whole months during our residency in Omaha. They just wanted their rent on the first of the month, come hell or high water.

Abigail's health seemed to improve over the next few months, and we settled into a routine with her appointments and mine. She saw her pediatrician in Lincoln every 28 days, where she received her dose of Synagis to keep the RSV bug away; she also had regular appointments with her neurosurgeon in Omaha. I saw my physical therapist and orthopedic surgeon regularly and healed as well as could be expected. I knew I would always have pain and ongoing issues from my injuries, especially with my neck, right shoulder, and right wrist. Because these injuries involved soft tissue damage, it was unlikely I would heal totally of those tears and strains. My bruises, cuts, and scrapes would eventually heal and my chipped teeth were filed off nicely by my dentist, ridding me of my temporary snaggle-toothed smile. Abi and I were on the road to recovery, albeit a long, mountainous one.

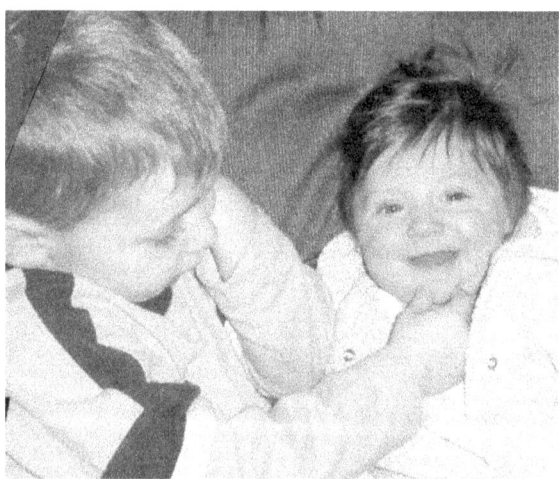

Abigail still was unable to go anywhere outside of the home besides her medical appointments, making family outings impossible. Brian and I were back to taking turns for grocery runs and errands to keep Abi safe from illness or infection. It was tricky and far from fun, but for the next four months, until spring had sprung, we were committed to keeping her out of the elements and safe from the outside world.

Noah was in awe of his new baby sister and tried his best to convert her into an admirer of cars like her big brother. Holding her brought him immense joy and he took his role as big brother quite seriously. He considered it his job to tell me what she was doing and what she wanted at all times, even though I was always right next to them both. Thinking back on the pride his new role brought him still makes me smile.

Back to Work

On January 13, 2003, I returned to work in Wahoo, which meant Brian and I had to find childcare for both children during business hours. Since taking Abi to a daycare facility at such a fragile time in her life could have been a death wish, we were left with no other choice than to search for a nanny. After interviewing several candidates, we finally hired a sweet young nanny who would be our temporary fix to a long-term problem. I went back to work excited at the idea of a reunion with my coworkers and with the prospect of restarting my career as a soil conservation technician. I had big plans for what I would accomplish, beginning with taking the soil classes that I needed to advance to a soil conservationist. Now that the pieces were slowly falling into place, I was a force to be reckoned with.

It felt incredible to be back at work, but I was distracted, to put it mildly. The nanny was great, but I longed to be the one to take care of my little ones instead of leaving them with a perfect stranger. I was torn every day thinking about how fortunate I was to have a job that I had worked my entire life to achieve, while simultaneously obsessing about what was happening at home in my absence. As time progressed, I was less torn and more worried about the chance that Abi could become sick again and I questioned whether the nanny would be able to handle such a huge amount of responsibility. Would she know if something was off one day? If she recognized that things were not as they should be, would she know what to do about it? Would she try to be a hero, or would she contact me or Brian with concerns?

Although I was back to working full-time hours, I still missed work regularly to get Abi to her appointments. I missed four full days during my third week back to work, and I struggled to focus on work while I was there, dealing with my own injury aftermath. Whatever the reason, my work life was under fire just as much as my personal life, and this lack of control was very scary to me.

There were always a million concerns and questions in the back of my mind, but I knew that I wanted and needed my job more than I could have described in words to anyone. I labored tirelessly to pay for school with one part-time job after another and applied everything I had to coursework for good grades to fulfill my dreams. I was laser-focused on my future in the environmental field and had the plan laid out to a T. I knew that I would graduate with my master's degree, go to work for the government in my field of study, and work to save the planet. I was not going to be thrown off course, not even by a near-fatal accident and a medically complex infant.

A Wrench in the Machine

One day in March, I received a fateful phone call from Brian. He almost never called me at work, and my heart immediately dropped when the office receptionist alerted me to the call. My mind went to dozens of places in the seconds that it took me to pick up the receiver, but every thought included Abi, not him. "Hello," I answered. His voice was calm as he began to fill me in on what had happened leading to the phone call. All I really remember is one short sentence: "I got fired." I thought he was joking. I thought that everything had fallen back into place for him after returning months before. There seemed to be little warning of such a possibility, rendering me utterly confused.

I quickly hurried home after notifying my ever-understanding supervisor; I could not possibly work the rest of the day with such a dark cloud looming overhead. Various thoughts raced through my mind as I sped from Wahoo to Lincoln. I prayed to God the entire 40 minutes that I was behind the wheel. I had a multitude of questions for Him, the biggest one being, "Why?" Hadn't we endured enough? I remember asking Him, "Just when I thought that we were pulling things together and recovering from the last catastrophe, You decided it was a good time to throw this our way?" A plethora of emotions flooded my entire being—I was angry, hurt, and hostile toward God. What could I have done that was so bad that it would have evoked such an accumulation of disastrous events? Little did I know, it was all just part of His plan, and it wasn't punishment for anything I had done. But at the time, it seemed like a cruel way to show me His love.

I frantically pulled into the driveway and made my way into the quiet duplex where Brian awaited my arrival. I listened to him tell me about the preceding week when his regional manager, the same one who promised to take special care of his branch while he tended to his injured wife and baby, wrote him up for poor performance. She gave him 90 days to turn the branch into the money maker that it was before the accident, stating if he couldn't make it happen by then, disciplinary action would be taken.

He was, of course, a bit caught off guard but knew that since life at home was settling down, he could give the branch his full attention. *No problem,* he thought. He had been working long hours and applying all that he had to his work and his employees, and he thought that his continued efforts could only prove beneficial for the company. One week later—far short of the 90 days she had promised—the same manager fired him because she became impatient. To make matters worse, Brian's company car was seized that day, and he was forced to hitch a ride home with her. When I heard that, I said, "I would rather walk 200 miles than get a ride from the person who fired me!" How humiliating!

Sitting around the dining room table after hearing his story, we devised a plan of attack where he would be unemployed for the shortest amount of time possible. I was confident he would throw his whole heart and soul into a new job search. Brian would have to find a job right away because my entry-level federal government salary would not come close to making ends meet. His salary at the car rental company was nearly three times as much as mine and our bank account would be taking a hit.

The next day was like any other for me. I greeted the nanny on my way out the door, as we planned to keep her employed while Brian was home job searching. Because we were optimistic that he would not be unemployed for long, we did not see a need to let her go. For a few days it worked out well; Brian stayed on the lowest level of the duplex working long hours sending out one resumé after another, while the nanny and children utilized the rest of the home as usual.

After about a week of this schedule, the nanny asked if she could come and pick me up for a soda, just the two of us. She said she needed to talk outside of the house in neutral territory and drove us to the nearby Sonic, where she proceeded to tell me that she was leaving. The situation was less than perfect for her (hell, it was less than perfect for all of us), as she felt Noah did not see her as a serious authority figure when Brian was home, which made her uncomfortable. I had no choice but to respect her decision. We were now without help, and taking care of Abigail and Noah was a full-time job.

Still, with the faith that God would never leave us stranded, we continued to clumsily stumble through each day, as humbled and needy as ever. After what seemed like an eternity of uncertainty, Brian was successful in landing a financial advisory position with a great company within a few weeks of losing his former job. There was only one thing to consider: Should we stay and continue to build a life for our family in Nebraska, or should we move back to Illinois where we possessed a strong support system of family and friends?

To learn more about the medical terms and topics discussed in this chapter, visit this link:

www.SavingAbigailGrace.com

CHAPTER SEVEN

Hometown Humble Pie

AFTER LEARNING OF BRIAN'S NEWLY acquired position, we had a major decision to make. Because the company was national, he had a choice between staying in Nebraska or moving back to Illinois. We made pros and cons lists and prayed that we would make the right decision for our family. We talked it over with my parents and other close confidants and struggled from one day to the next to finally decide. We needed to inform his new company of his intentions within the week, so after much thought and consideration, we decided it would be best to move back "home." After all, my parents and brothers lived in my hometown of Monmouth, and Brian's dad and his dad's wife were in Peoria, so it made sense to be where we thought we could get help when needed.

Because Brian would be studying from home for the first few months preparing for all the licensing exams he would soon take, we fortunately had some time to equip ourselves for the move while waiting for our lease to expire at the end of May. Reluctantly, I gave my supervisor my two-weeks' notice on May 12. I struggled through the remaining workdays, anxiously anticipating the end of my dream job, where I would leave behind many incredible coworkers and friends who had become my family.

Just as the idea of a new move was settling in, life threw us another curve ball and Abi landed in the emergency room.

Just three days after I gave my notice at work, Abi spiked a high fever, was vomiting, and was incredibly irritable, causing worry that her shunt may be malfunctioning. Following the instructions her neurosurgeon had given us prior to her last hospital release, I called their office for further guidance. Since fever and nausea were indicators of a shunt malfunction or infection, I was instructed with urgency to rush her to the Children's Hospital ER in Omaha, where—you guessed it— she would be admitted once again.

For the next three and a half days, we sat by her bedside in a place we knew all too well and waited patiently for answers. The sterile hospital smell had strangely become almost soothing to me, as did the beeps and hums of the equipment that made up the PICU at Children's Hospital. Upon admission, the neurology team tapped her shunt to draw a sample of the cerebrospinal fluid. They ran the fluid through a gamut of tests and performed cultures to determine whether there was a presence of bacteria or other microorganisms that may have caused her ill health. They also drew blood samples, hoping to rule out infection. Although the blood cultures showed presence of cocci (a bacterium), there was no sign of sepsis, and the conclusion for the moment was that she had a possible viral illness.

Abi was released on May 18, and I returned to work the following day, drained and a bit shaken. I wondered when we would be free of the constant fear that always seemed to linger. I wasn't a new parent and had experienced episodes of illness with Noah before, but I was new at parenting a newborn with preexisting conditions. Each time she became ill, I felt like Alice in Wonderland falling into a world of the unknown. I found it nearly impossible to let my guard down. How could I, given what we had already experienced?

Nevertheless, I made it through my last week of work and on my last day, May 23, 2003, I was both saddened at the thought that I might never be able to replicate my experience with the NRCS, and relieved that I could now focus on my sickly baby girl and her big brother. As I said my goodbyes, the tears came uncontrollably because I knew I had found something special with that job and the group of people that came with it. I had established such a history with them already; after all, they were the ones who witnessed the fateful crash on October 17, 2002, and they were the first ones on the scene that day. They were also the ones whose generosity proved to be abundantly significant to my family because of their donated PTO dollars. My family could not have made it through this situation financially had it not been for their unbelievable selflessness. They were often the sunshine on my darkest days, and they knew my struggles better than anyone. I would miss them more than I could even know at the time.

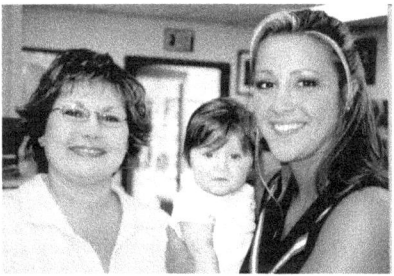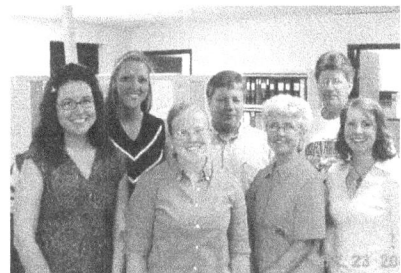

My incredible NRCS coworkers

Relocating

With Abi out of the hospital, we were ready for change. Moving day arrived five days later, hitting us like a ton of bricks. We packed up the U-Haul truck as we had done many times before, buckled the babies into their car seats, said goodbye to yet another city, and traveled that long stretch of I-80 through Nebraska, Iowa, and finally into Illinois. Brian and I both had mixed emotions about the move, since we had become attached to the city we had thought would be our final home. The mood was heavy, and our hearts were once again broken. Despite this, we were ready to greet the next chapter of our lives and were hopeful that all the dark clouds would stay in Nebraska.

Late springtime in the Midwest is a magical time, and the scenery along the highways can be breathtaking if you allow yourself to breathe it all in. With Noah and Abi passed out in the backseat, I had over eight hours to watch the rolling hills of corn and bean fields speckled with the brilliant yellows of goldenrod and perfect purples of deadnettle and henbit pass by. The skies were a vivid blue and created a picturesque backdrop for the trees, their bright green leaves softly swaying in the light breeze that the traffic created. With the dark thoughts temporarily escaping my mind, I sought solace in the pillowy white clouds that hung delicately in the sky and found myself searching for the pictures in them like I did when I was a kid lying in the grass. I was at peace.

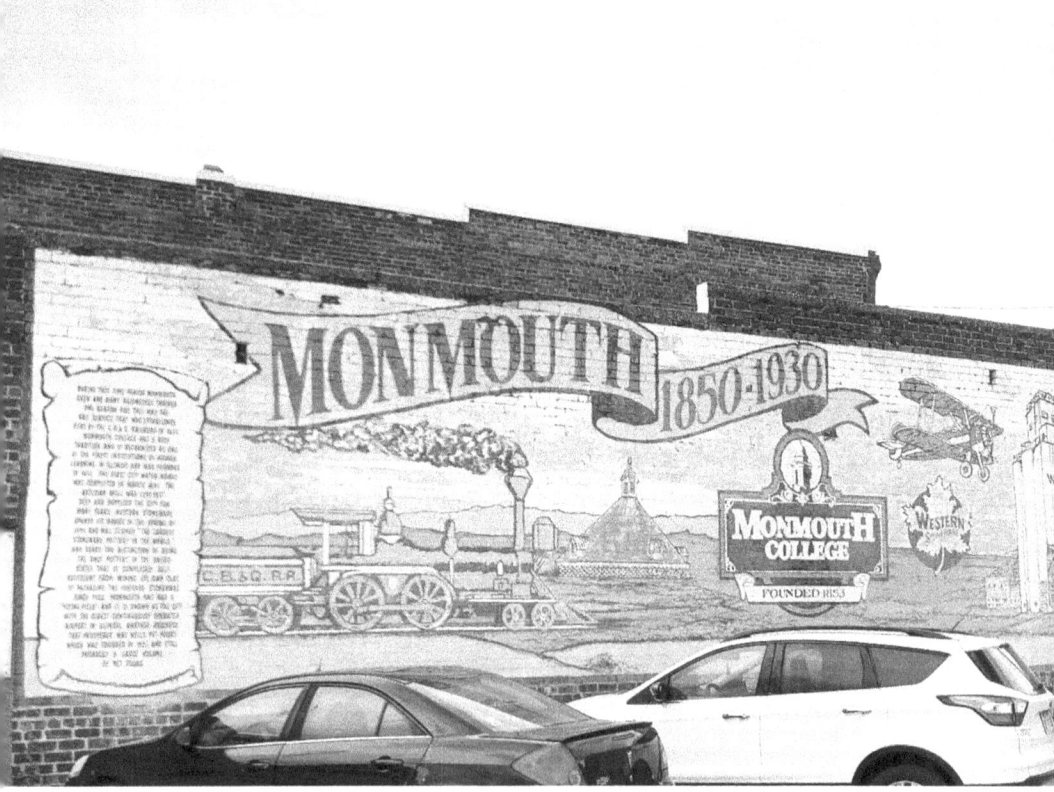

On Wednesday, May 28, 2003, we arrived in Monmouth, the town I would once again call my home, where our young family of four was confined to a tiny bedroom in my parents' house. It was the room that belonged to my mom and dad when I was growing up, but now it was just an empty room where we could lay our heads until our situation became more stable. It was great to see our welcoming crew who were eager to help us get unpacked and settled. Mom, Dad, and my brothers, Nathan and Gabriel, were at the house and, as soon as I saw them, it was as if all the yuck dripped from my body, replaced with hope and contentment.

My mom and dad were incredibly inviting and understanding of our needs with such a fragile seven-month-old baby, and they never missed a beat when it came to assisting in her care. Mom, being a nurse at the local hospital, had some knowledge of the delicate state in which Abigail existed. She was careful to let me be Mom while offering her unconditional help whenever it was needed, and it was vital in putting me at ease. My parents were instrumental during this time of healing and I'm not sure what I would have done without their support.

PTSD

With the support of my family, one would assume that I would feel a heavy burden lifted, but I often felt like I was walking a tightrope, and that at any moment I might plunge to my metaphorical death. I slowly found myself slipping into an undeniable state of depression and I was diagnosed with post-traumatic stress disorder (PTSD), a condition that affects an estimated 12 million Americans. Years of future therapy would teach me that because I was in "fight or flight" mode immediately following the accident and was deeply involved in fighting for my and my daughter's health, I pushed through the trauma until my brain decided I no longer needed to.

Even though I had help from my family, the stress would fester and build like a pimple that needed to pop. I dealt with my anxious feelings the only way I knew how: by staying busy—cleaning the house and caring for my children—while my parents were at work and my husband locked himself in our room to study. I didn't know then how much I could benefit from therapy, and I wouldn't let myself add appointments with a counselor into our already packed schedule, but eventually I would have to face the demons that were working overtime inside my brain.

After just a week in Monmouth, I headed to Illinois' capital city to take the exams needed to be considered for employment with the Environmental Protection Agency (EPA), a dream I'd had for more than a decade. Suffice it to say, I never did end up working for the EPA, and hindsight being what it is, I can now say that I am glad I didn't. God's plan prevailed over mine again, and I finally left that "dream" in the past.

With most of our belongings housed in a storage unit, we began planning Noah's third birthday party, which would also serve as a welcoming party to be attended by all of our closest Illinois friends and family. Saturday, June 7, 2003, was a glorious, heartfelt day celebrated by all, and Noah had such a great time with all of his new loot. He was still too young to understand the mess in which we had landed, and I am quite thankful for that. I'd like to think that he was never really affected by the turbulent events that led us to my parents' small-town backyard that day. I supposed only time would tell.

The following Monday morning, after my mom and dad had both headed in different directions to their workplaces, and after Brian had disappeared behind the door of our loaner bedroom to study, I began to desperately search for employment of my own. In the 29 years that I had spent in this crazy world, I could not remember ever being so stressed out and preoccupied with our financial situation. This was also the first time since I started babysitting neighbors' kids at the age of 12 that I had been un-employed. Add to that all the stress of the road ahead—taking Abi to one appointment after another with a new pediatrician, pediatric neurosurgeon, and therapists—and it was a recipe for utter exhaustion and crippling pressure.

I did the best I could, taking each day as it came and greeting it with prayers to God to help me through it all. His Word told me that He would never leave me, nor forsake me, and I was hanging onto that idea for dear life. I grew closer to Him than ever throughout this experience, and held Him to His Word all day, every day. What a blessing it was to be able to talk to God any time I pleased, knowing that He was always listening.

Trying to Acclimate

Since Brian, Noah, Abi, and I had all established doctor/patient relationships in Nebraska and needed to begin new relationships in Illinois, I spent a solid week filling out medical releases and writing letters to each facility. In 2003, we were still doing this with paper, pen, and a fax machine—can you imagine? This proved especially tricky and time-consuming for Abigail and me because we had seen several physicians and specialists after the accident. Of course, back then it was a bit different than it is now. Each facility needed a signed letter mailed to them with the appropriate signatures and specific requests for each set of records. Abigail had records in eight different locations, and my records were housed in six facilities. Between the writing involved in the medical records request process and the employment application process alone, I was quite busy!

Meanwhile, Brian and I worked together to fight the denial of his unemployment claim. I am sure you will not be surprised to hear that they took their time informing us— after completing all the appropriate paperwork and waiting for weeks—of the denial. The reason? Brace yourself: We learned that his former employer misrepresented the details of his termination to the Department of Employment Security. This was the drop that made the barrel run over. We'd both had it!

They say, "When it rains, it pours," and I was beginning to look for the Ark! We were drowning, and once again it became a very dark time for us. I was unemployed, Brian was newly employed but earning a very small salary while studying for his licensing exams, and now we were denied unemployment benefits. All we could do was continue to trust that everything would work out in God's perfect timing and keep our fingers crossed that His schedule was at least somewhat in line with ours. But even those with the greatest faith will, at some point, feel hopeless and have difficulty finding the silver lining.

Mom and Dad supported us in every way they could, but they were not exactly growing a money tree in their backyard either. Both earned an honest wage for hard work and did their best to manage their money responsibly, but they never really had a savings account, and "mad money"—or disposable income—was not a familiar term. Still, they were our earthly saviors during our most desperate time of need, offering help with the kiddos and never asking for us to pay our share of living expenses.

Although we found invaluable assistance from my parents while staying in their home, it was not meant to be our final stop. So, on Sunday, July 27, 2003, we moved into a rental home in an affordable but crime-filled part of Peoria, about an hour and a half drive from Monmouth. Since all our physicians and medical team members were affiliated with the Children's Hospital of Illinois in Peoria, we immediately began bouncing our way from one office to the next like kernels in a popcorn machine. I saw my general practitioner the day after we moved our belongings into our rental and hit the ground running. My body and mind had some healing to do, and it was finally time to start that process now that Abigail was no longer confined to her sterile hospital settings.

While I was busy making appointments to meet all of Abigail's new providers, sending in countless resumes, and dealing with the hearings for our case against the employment security office, I was also enduring horrific upper body pain that seemed to worsen as I became increasingly stressed. The aftermath of the accident left me with soft tissue damage in my right wrist, right shoulder, and neck, resulting in a constant state of pain and discomfort. Because of the tension in my neck and shoulder, I suffered from excruciating headaches that did not respond to any pain medication, unless you want to count the ones that knocked me out. I began seeing a chiropractor nearly every day to break up the scar tissue causing tightness in my wrist and shoulder, which finally brought me some relief.

We began the process of settling into yet another incredible chapter and welcomed new opportunities to grow in our faith. We had a new rental home to unpack and decorate, Brian had passed his licensing exams and was now pounding the pavement in search of clients, and I was earning my unofficial title of caregiver in every way imaginable.

Most days consisted of unpacking a few boxes and putting belongings away room by room, scheduling and carting the children to various appointments, feeding, bathing and caring for the kiddos once we were back home, packing everyone up for another appointment, putting Abi and Noah down for their naps, and, in my "free time," sending off resumes in search of employment.

Although we needed the income, I was skeptical as to how I would pull off being a full-time employee while holding down the fort at home. These were the days before working remotely became common. Because Brian was still in training mode at his new job, his travel time away from home was significant, leaving me to be a single parent for up to a week at times. If I were to become employed, I would need to hire someone to handle Abi's appointments, making a meaningful salary a necessity.

Both children would be members of the daycare society, which wasn't free by any stretch of the imagination. The thought of being a stay-at-home mom was one that would have never occurred to me in my previous life. After all, I had dreamed of and planned every detail of my career path and was determined not to be derailed, no matter what mountains stood in my way!

My schedule had become so jam-packed that the decision about work was made almost entirely for me: I would not return to work for the time being and would instead become the one thing I had worked diligently to avoid becoming—a stay-at-home mom. The funny thing about that term is that I was nothing of the sort, not unlike most other moms. Staying at home was something I only wished I could do at times. Overwhelmed and frantic for the better part of each day, I found myself quickly choking down not just a slice of but an entire humble pie.

Even though Brian was working out of our home office—which was nothing more than a cleared-off spot on the dining room table—I could not rely on him for help if I wanted him to be successful at his job. He was left to plug away and come and go as needed to bring home the only paycheck we were relying on. There was no way I could return to work, and that was something I had to learn to accept. I would later come to understand, after fighting it every step of the way, that this was exactly how God intended it.

Since making the move from my parents' house in Monmouth, our so-called support system had all but disintegrated. Although Brian's dad and his dad's wife lived in the same town as us, we rarely saw them or any of Brian's siblings, who also lived nearby. If there was ever a need for someone to stay with the children, we would be forced to hire a sitter. I found it ironic that we based our decision to move from Nebraska on the idea of having more support in Illinois, yet no one seemed to have the time or the desire to help when we needed it. During this period of my life, I learned who I could and could not depend upon for support and assistance—and many family members ended up on the "could not" list.

Because Noah had been outside the routine of a social environment since the accident occurred nearly one year ago, Brian and I decided that it would benefit him to attend preschool regularly. After all, he was now three years old and needed to be actively learning what children his age should know—things like how to behave around peers, how to share with others, and the knowledge to be gained from books. Up to this point, I had done my best to keep him on track with his ABCs and 123s, but I was not a teacher. In fact, I knew he was missing out on constructive play with friends. On Thursday, September 4, Noah ventured into a new world of books, glue sticks, and glitter.

Noah was more ready to attend school than I was to let him go. Naturally, I had become very protective of my little family and worried every second that I was away from my kiddos, so dropping him off that first day was tough. He made friends easily, just like his dad always had, and he stepped through the classroom doors without giving me a second glance. As I made my way back to my vehicle with Abi hanging from my left arm in her carrier, I was filled with mixed emotions—sad that it seemed so easy for Noah to leave me, excited for him to meet new friends and experience new things, and somewhat relieved that I would be able to accomplish my daily goals without the hundreds of interruptions that came from having a toddler underfoot, which also made me feel guilty.

After a short time, we had become established in our new roles and routines and seemed to be on cruise control. Brian was committed to his new role as a financial advisor and doing well to accommodate his new clients. I was settling into this so-called stay-at-home-mom thing, wearing the hats of teacher, caregiver, taxi service, maid, accountant, and countless others. Abigail was making progress in her therapy sessions, her health was improving, and she even seemed to be slowly catching up to her peers developmentally. By then, she had her first tooth, was crawling, and keeping me very busy with her constant curiosity. Before long, it would be her first birthday, a celebration filled with a variety of emotions, but a celebration nonetheless. Our first year would be behind us, and we would look ahead, hoping to see a road paved with happy memories, in contrast to the dark and uncertain path we had traveled.

To learn more about the medical terms and
topics discussed in this chapter, visit this link:

www.SavingAbigailGrace.com

CHAPTER EIGHT

Doctors, Specialists, and Therapists, Oh My!

THE DAUNTING TASK IN FRONT of me was to locate the necessary physicians and specialists and make appointments with them all. Abi's neurosurgeon in Omaha referred us to one in Peoria, and on June 10, 2003, when Abi was nearly eight months old, we met her new pediatric neurosurgeon for the first time. A small, gentle, quiet man, he was a stark contrast to her original neurosurgeon—a tall, lean man who pulled no punches. Upon examination, he noted a left-sided weakness but never elaborated on it and made note that the shunt was a bit sluggish. Other than that, we had no new information and were scheduled for a routine follow-up appointment on our way out the door. In the meantime, she would have a CT scan of her head to determine whether the shunt was functioning properly to prevent cerebrospinal fluid from building pressure on her brain. In addition, they would take X-rays of her head and torso for what they called a "shunt series." That would show the mechanical portion of the shunt, its cord, and the condition of the entire system. The two scans would give the specialists an unmistakable idea of the overall functionality of Abi's shunt, thereby gauging her hydrocephalus from the most favorable perspective.

After researching pediatricians in hopes of finding one who was well trained in hydrocephalus and knowledgeable of gadgets such as VP shunts, I found a talented doctor who would prove a great choice for many years to come.

The pediatrician checked Abigail thoroughly and made note of his findings, expanding on a term that we hadn't heard since we left Nebraska but would quickly become familiar with: cerebral palsy (CP). I was just beginning to get acquainted with all the other terms that had branded her, and now this.

What is cerebral palsy?

According to a study published at the National Library of Medicine, cerebral palsy "is the most common motor disorder among children, affecting approximately 1 in 500 newborns." It is caused when there is interference in early (birth to 2 years of age) brain development—in Abi's case, traumatic brain injury that occurred in utero. Those who live with CP experience difficulty with voluntary muscular movement and increased spasticity, making it difficult to control motor movements. Although spasticity is a neuromuscular condition where the brain and nervous system do not communicate clearly, when treated early in a child's development, these motor movements can be improved. Later in this chapter, we will learn of treatments that have been proven to help CP patients. Cerebral Palsy Research Network is a great source to learn more about CP, how to diagnose it, and treatments that work.

When the pediatrician performed specific tests on Abigail for strength and agility in her appendages, he found that her left side was significantly weaker and more spastic than her right side. This information would parallel what was noted in our visit with the neurosurgeon only days before. I had noticed previously that she tended to favor her left arm and held it in an upright position, as if it were in a sling, but I never really gave it much thought. And since she was not yet walking or crawling, I hadn't realized that her left leg showed signs of the same.

Abi was still, after nearly three-quarters of a year, experiencing insufferable issues with her bowels. She had always experienced terrible discomfort with her infrequent bowel movements, and it never seemed to improve. On this particular day, she screamed in pain to every gentle push of her pediatrician's hands on her distended belly. What I found interesting in my research on CP was that chronic constipation can be quite common in people with the condition. The more I researched on my own, the more I discovered that many of Abi's ailments were deeply intertwined with her CP diagnosis—information that would come in handy as I explored treatment options for her.

Finally, adding to the already troubling list of ailments, her doctor seemed alarmed by the developmental motor delays that he observed. She was significantly behind other children her age in even the most basic categories, and I sensed a strong urgency in terms of getting her evaluated further.

With this newfound information, her doctor sent us home with a referral for both physical therapy (PT) and occupational therapy (OT) at a facility of my choice. My next step was to contact Easter Seals and Children's Hospital of Illinois and consider which one offered exactly what she needed.

As I navigated the process of making one phone call after another to various facilities and organizations, I discovered that the state of Illinois had an early intervention service. This service would come to our home and evaluate Abigail in her natural surroundings, while observing her perform a vast number of tasks given by a developmental therapist. This specialist evaluated Abi on a multitude of various skills such as social, adaptive, motor, communication, and cognitive skills, and then assigned a number for whether she expressed a delay in each. It was quite extraordinary to see all the tools that accompanied the specialist—tools that, to any nine-month-old, looked like a toy wonderland. If only Abi had been allowed to do what she wanted with them, she would have been a much happier camper! To say she was discouraged and exhausted by the end of her two-hour "play date" would be an understatement, but it would all prove incredibly beneficial for her evaluation.

Abi's New OTs/PTs

Upon completion of her evaluation for early intervention services, I was referred to a physical therapist, an occupational therapist, and a developmental therapist, all of whom were connected to Children's Hospital of Illinois. Immediately, appointments to evaluate her from each perspective were arranged, beginning with PT, then OT. With a delicate disposition, the therapists took Abi through a journey where she had tons of fun playing with colorful toys, some of which neither she nor I had ever seen. She was sometimes discouraged by some of the tasks that she was asked to do because they were hard work for her. I noticed that she would get irritated when her therapist asked her to use her left hand and fingers instead of her right. It got to the point where the adults would hold her right hand behind her back to force her through the exercises, making it quite an interesting task for us all.

Each therapist patiently observed her range of motion, muscle strength and tone, and gross and fine motor patterns. It took her more time to accomplish certain tasks using her left arm, hand, and fingers than it did when she used her right extremities. A 33 percent delay was noted in her grasping abilities. When she tried to grasp a small object such as a Cheerio, it was difficult for her to pick it up without dropping it. Grasp patterns were not typical for a child her age. She was uncomfortable using her left hand and fingers to pick up an object and would immediately transfer them to her right hand. Her coordination was underdeveloped, and she was extremely dependent upon others to help her perform tasks with her left side, such as feeding herself and grasping toys.

After the therapists finished evaluating Abi's abilities

through observation of specific play activities, they each wrote up their separate reports and recommendations. As I expected, both therapists found considerable motor delays in Abigail's development. The reports reflected much of what had already been discovered by Abi's physicians and specialists. Abigail showed up to a 30 percent delay in areas of grasping with her left upper extremity, visual motor integration skills with her left upper extremity, and muscle strength and tone on the left side. She also preferred to hold her left hand in the form of a fist and found it difficult to extend her fingers openly, due to increased muscle tone or spasticity on that side. This was typical of a child with cerebral palsy and could be improved with the appropriate physical and occupational therapy, thankfully.

The evaluations recommended starting regular developmental, physical, and occupational therapies to correct developmental delays.

Developmental therapy (DT) began on September 25, 2003, and was a weekly activity for Abi and me for almost a year. In a group setting, the goal was to "increase overall developmental skill progress through targeted play, routine schedules, and peer interaction," according to the therapist's notes. Abi had the privilege of being in a learning environment for an hour and a half session every Thursday

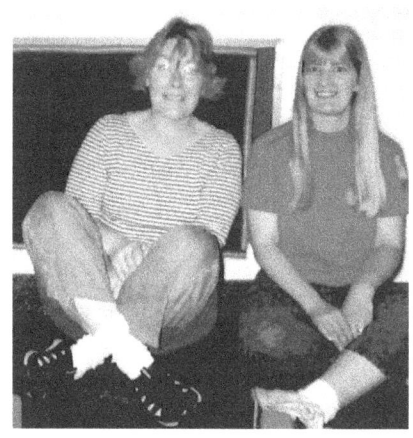

Abi's developmental therapists

morning, where she was surrounded by children with similar disabilities. In November 2003, we took the opportunity to attend DT every Tuesday and Thursday, doubling her time with the therapists. This proved to be a remarkable experience that enabled Abi to make profound improvements, and at the same time, opened permanent relationships for me with other parents and caregivers.

Abigail learned to use gestures and expressive language, interacting with children her age, and grew in her ability to play in a structured environment. This was all incredibly important for any child to learn and usually comes naturally, but for children with certain disabilities, it becomes imperative. Each session consisted of a greeting where we all sang a welcome song together, and then we went into circle time for a short period. During circle time, all the children, parents, caregivers, and therapists made a big inclusive circle where we did a fun group activity. After that, all of us moved over to the tiny tables and chairs where the children were each involved as a group in table activities like stacking blocks or matching items to their pictures on a sheet of paper. The activities were always fun and educational but proved challenging for Abigail at first, as they required using the right and left upper extremities simultaneously. It was a great deal of work for her and there were many tantrums at our table. It was a time of growing patience for both of us.

After the table activities, the group of kiddos was released for some "organized free play" (sounds like an oxymoron, I know), and much of the observation by the DTs would occur at this time. They watched for things such as peer interaction and modeling. The DTs also observed how and whether the children could share with one another during this play time. I recall the very beginning of these developmental therapy sessions and how most of the children had no concept of sharing, and many had no desire to play with any of their peers. Many times, a madhouse ensued during a time that should have been one of great fun and pleasure. It could be stressful for us parents who witnessed our children behave in ways that could be considered socially unacceptable. Because many of the kiddos did not yet understand how to express their emotions in acceptable ways, they would sometimes hit each other, snatch each other's toys aggressively, or break down in terrible tantrums. I caught myself wondering on occasion whether Abi would ever be able to behave appropriately in social situations. I could only hope and pray throughout the process that all would work out according to God's plan, having faith that it would—it had to!

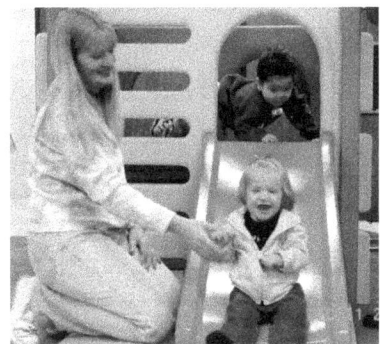 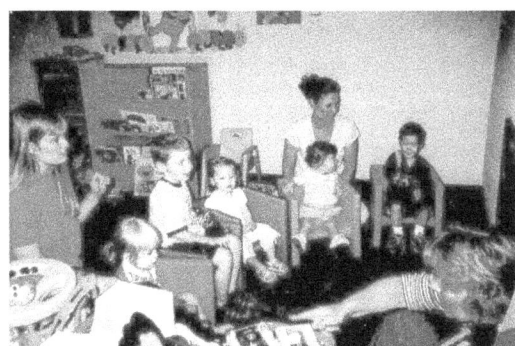

Physical therapy began one week earlier than DT and occurred once a month, each session lasting one hour. The focus of these sessions was to improve Abigail's use of her left side, in hopes of balancing it with the use of her right side. There was a series of activities each time we met with the PT—some fun for Abi and others which were total challenges met with great defiance. For an entire year, Abi powered through some obstacles and crumbled beneath others. We identified improvements and setbacks, and were encouraged and then hopeless, but the result was an overall progression. She and I also worked together at home on a series of stretches and exercises to strengthen her muscles. In September 2004, just shy of being two years old, Abigail was released from the PT program after showing notable progress.

December 10, 2003, was Abigail's first day with her OT, whom she would continue to see once a month for an hour-long session until September 2004. She was released upon achieving her goals of improvement in strength and awareness to the left extremity, use of the upper left extremity, grasp skills, transition skills, and visual motor integration skills. She also demonstrated appropriate follow-through of therapeutic activities, especially in her home exercise program.

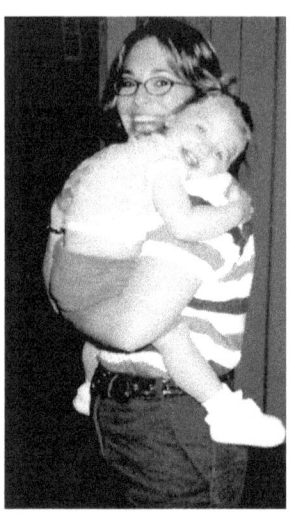

Abi and her occupational therapist

Each goal was reached by using weight-bearing activities such as those she naturally used by supporting herself in specific exercises and play. She also used a myriad of blocks, Lego pieces, and food items to build impressive towers, working with the pincers on each hand as equally as possible despite her left-sided weakness. After nine months of treatment with her occupational therapist, I was amazed at the progress she made and pleased when she transitioned into a home program, where I took on the roles of physical and occupational therapists, along with mom, nurse, and teacher.

Chiropractic Discovery and Relief

The entire time I was taking Abi to one therapy appointment after another, she was also seeing a chiropractor who was able to keep her tiny skeletal system in alignment, while manipulating her muscles to function properly. Dr. Joe, a long-time friend of Brian's, had become part of our family over the years, and successfully treated all of us. It was only natural that I trusted him to work with Abi in tandem with her various therapists. Towering at six foot four with dark skin and black hair, he was a giant to my tiny munchkin, which made watching him work on Abi quite extraordinary. I decided to have him take a comprehensive look at her when she was just beginning to sit up on her own, as I had noticed that she was unable to straighten her left leg.

Over a series of appointments, Dr. Joe worked carefully and skillfully to loosen the muscle tone in Abi's' leg, and one day out of the blue, she sat on the floor with both legs in a perfect V shape! It was miraculous to Dr. Joe and me, and we simultaneously shed tears of joy. From that point forward, I became a strong advocate of chiropractic care, and our entire family still sees Dr. Joe regularly.

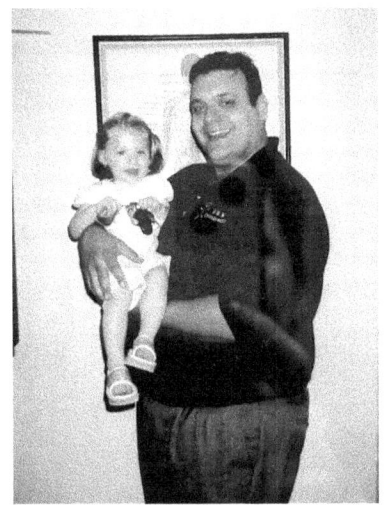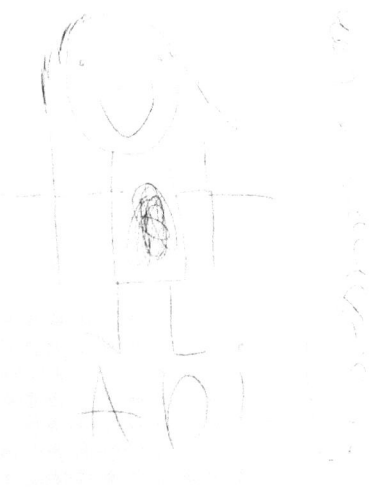

Abi with Dr. Joe and her drawing that still hangs in his office today

As time progressed, Abigail and I became increasingly comfortable with the relationships we were building with our healthcare providers, and we both were skipping along on our road to recovery. Although Abi was still developmentally behind other children her age, the gaps seemed to shrink with each day that passed, and I was encouraged to think that the dark days were behind us. Abigail began to crawl, and shortly after her first birthday, began to walk. It was at this point that we discovered the significance of her earlier CP diagnosis. Her left-sided weakness jumped the line in front of all of her other diagnoses. It suddenly wasn't just her left arm that put her behind in terms of physical development, but her left leg caused difficulty with her mobility. She was much more unstable on two legs than other children who were learning to walk, which meant her hard work was far from over.

Meanwhile, Brian was plugging along in his new job and

working countless hours to keep money in the bank and food on the table. I admired how focused he was on building a great book of business the only way he knew how—with self-determination and a plethora of elbow grease. He grew his clientele the old-fashioned way, by wearing holes in the soles of his wing tips and knocking on thousands of doors. As difficult as it was, he believed it was the only way to earn a living and the respect of his colleagues and clients.

Noah easily and quickly grew accustomed to his new school routine, sharing his daily happenings with us all when he got home in the afternoons. He behaved as if school was his job, and like daddy, he was doing his part to provide for us girls. It was heartwarming to witness how important it made him feel and how excited he was to give his reports over after school snacks or at the dinner table. Abi would stare at him in adoration as he baby-talked his way through a quick chat with her, making sure she had her favorite toys within reach, and then off he went into his room to perfectly line up his Matchbox cars.

A tip from Layla

Parents, talk to your pediatrician about early intervention services as soon as you notice anything about your child that may indicate delays in his or her development. The sooner they can be evaluated, the less precious time will be wasted. Early childhood development specialists suggest that the years between birth and three years of age can be the most important time for correcting delays.

CHAPTER NINE

Faith and Firsts

OVER THE NEXT SEVERAL YEARS, God took us on a roller coaster ride of ups and downs, ins and outs, teaching us to trust in Him and growing in our faith. Abi experienced periods of good health, only to be knocked down and dragged in and out of hospitals and medical facilities. Just when we found ourselves in comfort and peace, we knew to brace ourselves for turbulence ahead. It kept us on our toes and kept me in a state of emotional confusion, exacerbating my depression.

Since moving back to Peoria, we had once again become regular attendees at the Baptist church where we were members. It was like therapy in the beginning, and I dove in headfirst. I sang in the choir, Brian and I assisted as leaders in teaching Sunday school for the teens, we were involved in a Bible study where we were both students and teachers, as well as a biblical financial class. Our family attended church services every Wednesday and Sunday evening, Sunday school before service on Sunday morning, and Bible studies on Monday nights. If the doors were unlocked, we were there.

The church had been good to us while we were away in Nebraska, and our pastors were instrumental in coaching me through the dark days in Abi's NICU room via telephone. I learned a great deal about my relationship with God and with other Christians and relied heavily upon those relationships.

Also indispensable during that time was my Bible, which I clung to at all hours of the day.

Now that Abigail was walking, we were confronted with a series of questions, concerns, and more appointments with specialists. Because the CP affected her left side only, Abi was out of balance when she walked, causing her to be considerably clumsy. Her left leg did not have the same strength as her right, often causing her to fall, leaving her with scrapes and bruises on her legs and arms. She became cautious as she cruised along in the early days, and I was just as hesitant to watch her perform even the simplest of tasks because I hated to watch her tumble.

After consulting with doctors, we obtained a referral to have her fitted for a brace that she wore on her left leg. It served as a stabilizer, and the hope was that she would be able to strengthen her muscles and loosen the spasticity in her leg through exercises and stretches. Thanks to her PT, who provided us with loads of activities to do in our home program, she was able to work through this slowly. Over the years, we saw that the left-sided weakness was an obstacle in many physical activities. Riding a bike and swimming would prove particularly difficult for her.

Our First House

Because we were living in a rental house, we decided to begin looking for a more permanent housing solution. In January 2004 we contacted a real estate agent and got serious about finding a home to call our own. Being first-time home buyers, we were a bit naive about the process and learned quickly that buying a home was an extensive process, time consuming, and frustrating at times. During our home search, our landlord informed us that someone had bought the house we were living in, and we would have to move. So, on March 27, we moved out of the rental house and into a church friend's home that had only recently become vacant. The timing was perfect as they needed someone to rent it for a short time while they were transferred to the missionary field.

This house was in a more kid-friendly neighborhood than the last one, although it still was not what we desired at the time. We continued our search as home buyers, dedicating many Saturdays to house hunting with our agent. One day, we stumbled upon a subdivision just outside of Peoria city limits that we hadn't known about before, and thought it might be a great place to call home while the children were tiny tots. The homes had been built in the late 1960s/early 1970s and needed updating. Most of the homes we had walked through boasted original decor, appliances, and amenities, which meant extra costs to bring them into the 21st century. After looking at half a dozen homes in the subdivision, we found one that was in our price range and decided to make an offer.

We reached a major milestone on July 23, 2004, becoming homeowners for the first time. On August 1, at the age of 30, Brian and I moved with our two children, who were four and nearly two years old, into our new home. We were elated at the reality of finally being permanent residents of a single-family dwelling. Since we began dating eight years prior, we lived in seven different homes located in five different cities and two different states.

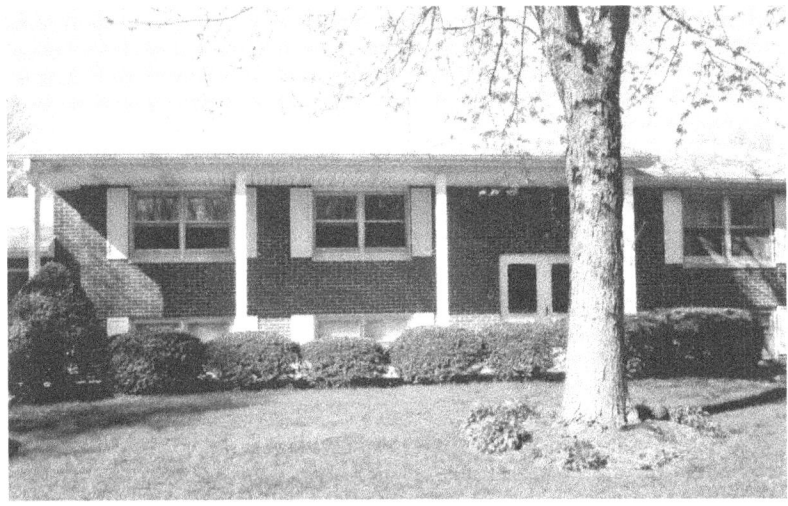

Our first home

The timing could not have been more perfect. It was summertime, Noah would begin preschool soon, and now that we were established in a new district, he would be able to attend a great school in a school district that was more aligned with our children's needs. We were finally achieving what we had always wanted for ourselves, the red brick home with a white picket fence and a bus stop at the end of the drive in a safe, middle-class neighborhood. It was glorious!

A New Business for Brian

Now that we were settled into our permanent residence, Noah was going to preschool and Abi was gaining momentum, while I was finally starting to get comfortable in this new life. But Brian was still struggling to earn the kind of money that he knew financial advisors could make and was becoming restless in his ventures. He resented not being involved in the daily happenings with the children, and missing many of Abi's appointments, so we began to discuss options for making a better living together.

A decision that seemed to come out of nowhere for me was one that Brian had mulled over for quite some time. He decided to leave the demands of his current employer and open a flooring installation business of his own. After a lot of discussion, I was to become the business manager who wore a number of different hats, including accounts payable and receivable, human resources, bookkeeping, and client relations.

The idea of being a small business owner was possibly even scarier for me than being involved in another life-altering vehicular crash. I could not fathom taking on that responsibility on top of the already full plate in front of me. A consistent paycheck was a necessity for me, and to leave that behind for an inconsistent, sometimes nonexistent, payday was terrifying.

I had been working odd jobs during the evenings to provide some income to supplement Brian's and was far from happy about it, but it was working for us. I waited tables at several restaurants and worked as a cocktail waitress at a few downtown

Peoria establishments to make ends meet. At the time, it seemed to be the only way I could earn a paycheck while having my days free to take care of the children. Even though Noah was in school, it was only during the afternoon for about three hours, and Abi's care was a full-time job on its own. With Brian's hectic work schedule and occasional need to be out of town during the week (we had to take all the work we could get, which often meant working in other states), I was again living the life of a single parent. Unless I wanted to hire a full-time caregiver—where would that money come from considering my money tree was bare?—I had no other choice but to continue working evening jobs. With the creation of the business, I would certainly see no end to this routine of hustling like I was a college student again.

To top it off, I was worried about losing insurance. Individual health insurance for Brian, Noah, and me bore an astronomical price tag and since no insurer would touch Abi with a 10-foot pole, we were forced to get state-provided Medicaid insurance for her. Since the state of Illinois had been known to not pay their bills, medical providers included, not all providers were willing to see patients with this type of health insurance.

But no matter how scared I was, my entrepreneurial-minded husband was determined to make it work and in October 2004, we began operating our new flooring/decorative concrete installation business together. Brian had it all figured out—he would have more flexibility in his workdays, allowing him to be more present in Abi's care and to attend her appointments. He would also be able to earn an honest living doing much of what he was already doing in his financial advisory position. The responsibility of finding clients and marketing the business would initially be his, but I would work that responsibility into my daily chores eventually. Because he was detail-oriented and creative, working in home and business interiors was a perfect outlet for him.

As a teenager, Brian cut his teeth, so to speak, on ceramic tile installation working for his grandfather, Dale. Dale owned a ceramic tile installation company that his father founded in 1922 and made an honorable name for himself in the business. Like many of the Slater men, Brian had gained incredible skills by working alongside his perfectionist grandfather and was troubled by the fact that, since the passing of his grandmother in 1990, the company had fallen dormant.

After discussing his ideas with his grandfather, Brian decided to build on the company that had existed successfully for nearly 70 years by adding other elements such as decorative concrete. Brian was trained to install various decorative applications of concrete by his brother-in-law, Doug, who owned a similar business in southern California with Brian's sister, Tammy. Their experience was amazing considering that they worked with high-end clients in the Los Angeles and Beverly Hills areas. Tammy was instrumental in helping me, as I had no idea how to run a business, and she taught me how to use QuickBooks to manage everything money-related. We worked as a team with our California relatives and learned from each other over the course of the next five years. It was quite a well-oiled machine, and it served our needs just fine, as our relationship with Tammy, Doug, and their three girls had always been solid and supportive.

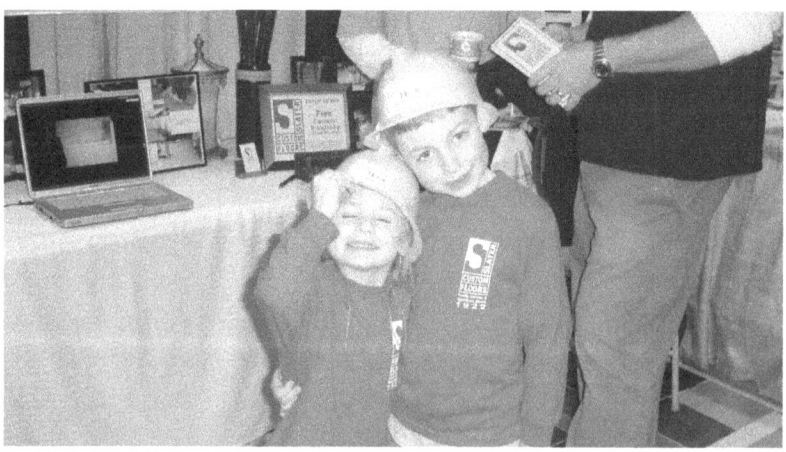

The kiddos representing our brand at the Peoria Home Show

Although Brian was more available to our family most of the time, he would still find himself traveling more than we had originally anticipated. He flew to California on many occasions to assist Doug with big jobs and to learn new skills and applications. In turn, Doug would fly to Peoria when Brian needed a skilled set of hands. They worked well together, and Doug taught Brian a great deal about the trade that proved valuable and irreplaceable. I don't know what we would have done without them!

Our First Big Contract

Almost immediately, after an intense process of bidding for the job and tough negotiating, we landed a huge contract with a well-known corporate client. As a result, we were able to employ a good number of friends and family members who were unemployed at the time. We were amazed and in awe of the complexity of the job that was a total remodel of an existing grocery store. Our company was hired to tear out the old flooring and install a common VCT. The materials were expensive, and we did not have the means to purchase them before being paid for work to be performed, so to make this job a reality, we had to do two terrifying things: we maxed out our line of credit with the bank, and reluctantly borrowed money from a friend who was also a small business owner with liquid cash.

The job was in a town about two hours from Peoria. Besides the cost of materials, there were many expenses to consider, as the crew would not always be traveling back and forth. We could have (and in hindsight, should have) walked away from it, but if things were to go as planned, we would have a great experience to add to our résumé, as well as a healthy profit.

As you may have already guessed, things didn't work out as we planned, and our client handed us our very first punch in the gut as a new installer. Not only did we receive no deposit from this multi-million-dollar company, but we also didn't get a single penny. After going into debt up to our eyeballs with the bank and with our friend, we found ourselves in a deep, dark pit that we would spend the next four years fighting and clawing to climb out of.

While we were battling it out in court to get what was rightfully ours from our first big client, we continued to build our business in the best way that we could. We worked with a multitude of residential and corporate clients and gave them our genuine attention. After a few years, we were finally earning paychecks comparable to what we earned while working in Nebraska. I learned valuable lessons and skills, while discovering traits about myself I never knew existed. Who would have known that I could actually succeed at being a small business owner? Had it not been for the dark cloud of debt always hovering, we could have really made something of the business, but we just could not seem to recuperate from that first terrible blow. Although we pursued a lawsuit against our client and chased the enormous invoice for years in vain, in the end, we would ultimately pay with our livelihood. We closed the business in 2009 with nothing to show for it except a jaded outlook on our legal system and a mountain of corporate debt.

Doing What Needs to Be Done

In July 2005, less than one year after starting our flooring business, my former boss asked me to rejoin the team of environmental health practitioners as a temporary part-time employee at the health department where I worked before moving to Nebraska. This was yet another way that I could earn additional money to improve our situation, but it was incredibly difficult to juggle that position with the responsibilities I had at our own company. On days when I was scheduled at the health department, I had to transfer our business phones to Brian's cell phone, and he would have to play receptionist as he installed materials at various job sites. It was far from a perfect system, but we did what we had to do to make ends meet.

One thing I appreciated about the 40-minute commute to and from my job at the health department was the alone time it allowed me with Abi in the car. With Noah in preschool, I took Abi to the YMCA where the staff looked after her while I was at work. Being around other kiddos her age helped her further sharpen her social skills, and she made friends, particularly with one little girl named Sloan. She called her "Sloanie Balonie," likely because that was the fun nickname the teachers gave her.

I also continued to plug away at night waiting tables and serving cocktails, just as I had before we decided to open the business. Between juggling the roles of part-time small business owner and environmental health practitioner by day, waitress by night, and handling my anything-but-typical mommy duties, I was slowly beginning to lose myself.

I still had not fully recovered mentally from the accident and all the wreckage it brought into my life. Before opening the business, I saw a therapist to help me disassemble all my negative emotions, only to reassemble them into something more positive. We came up with a plan of how I would overcome the PTSD with which I was diagnosed. I don't know whether it really helped or not, but I did what I was told to do by completing homework assignments and making lists to sort through my ever-changing feelings. I was skeptical to begin with, so I'm sure my negative attitude did nothing to help my healing, and since I didn't feel I had the time to dedicate to therapy, I finally gave up the metaphorical ghost.

The Strains of Life Changes

Reflecting, I can now see that I focused so much on Abi's care and fitting in professionally wherever I could find a place, that I became an amoeba of sorts—a chameleon blending perfectly into my circumstances, with no true identity of my own. Since the day Brian and I became a serious couple, I followed him where his jobs took him, placing my own dreams on hold, time and time again. Although I was the one with the advanced degree and huge career aspirations, I was somehow also the one forced to leave those plans in the rearview mirror with each of Brian's promotions and job changes. Over time, I built a tall wall of resentment between the two of us that was only occasionally penetrable.

If I haven't already demonstrated how much I crave control in my life, this is where it may become quite clear. My entire existence from the day I was born was built on being an independent woman, no matter the age. I was stubborn as a child and made my own choices, regardless of what my parents wanted for me, because I always knew who I was and what I could offer others. Self-confidence was not a trait I usually lacked, and I was never afraid to be different from the other girls if it meant I was remaining true to myself. I was most comfortable in the driver's seat, and as I zoomed out of the current map of my life where I could look at it with a bird's eye view, I saw myself as only a passenger.

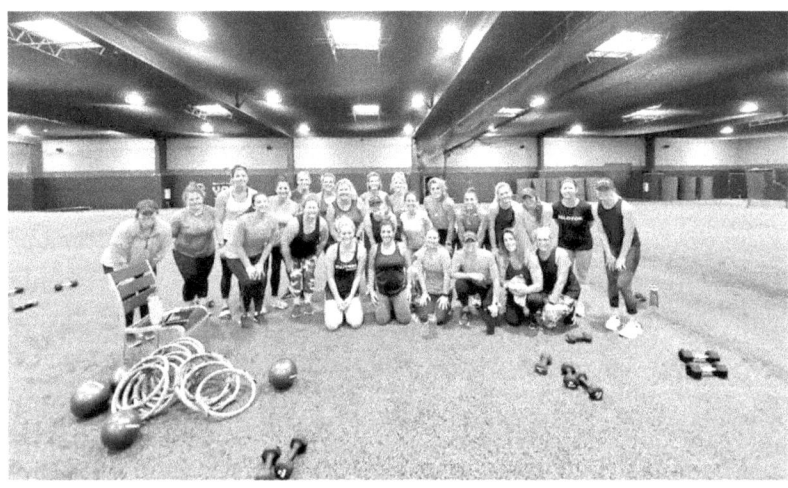

Me with my Sculpt Mode class

All I could do was make the best of my circumstances and take control of wherever I needed it most. I adapted, just like Charles Darwin taught in his theory of natural selection. I know—you're thinking, *Layla, you're a Christian; how can you be referencing Darwin?* It's as simple as this important concept which I encourage everyone to embrace: survival of the fittest.

Life is fluid, my friends, and if you do not adapt, you do not survive. And if your goal in life is to not only survive but to thrive, you must adapt. You must adapt with each experience—whether it's a positive, negative, or indifferent— so that's what I did, and that's what I continue to do.

A Pep Talk

Although it may not always be socially acceptable, it is normal for those of us who experience any kind of trauma to go into survival mode for a bit. Many times, and with as far as women have come in American culture, it is more often the woman whose dreams suffer. It is in our innate DNA to nurture and to care for our children and for our spouses, focusing on others and deserting our own needs and desires while doing so. We pick up all the loose ends that may become unraveled, while our male counterparts go to work and earn a living, as they have been taught to do. If you aren't aware that this will likely happen and take no steps to acknowledge it, you may lose sight of your dreams as your new job of caregiver takes the wheel of this tumultuous journey, increasing the odds of realizing it only after it is too late to change it.

This has happened to me many times throughout my journey. As I sit in front of my computer typing these words, I am only now fully aware that, over 20 years after my life-changing accident, I am still searching for my own identity. Therefore, I want to offer some advice in the hopes that it might help: communicate with your spouse, seek professional help when necessary, and allow yourself to do something—no matter how small—that brings you joy and has absolutely nothing to do with any-one else's needs.

What works for me may not work for everyone, but I find that when I am wandering around in a cloud of self-doubt or stagnancy, moving my body and exercising my mind in new ways feels magical. Whether it's dancing to your favorite music, taking yoga, Pilates, or barre classes, or slamming heavy weights around in a sweaty gym, physical activity can help clear a cluttered mind. Speaking of the mind, I believe exercising your brain is equally as important as physical exercise. Some of my favorite activities include taking a new art class like pottery, drawing, painting, or jewelry making. If you want to explore the art of words, take a creative writing class, learn to write poetry, or maybe just read the words of others in books.

I also find incredible joy in helping others, and there is never a shortage of nonprofit organizations that need help. Seek organizations that speak to your heart and find ways to give back. If you love animals, reach out to a local shelter or zoo to volunteer. People always need food, so consider calling a local food bank, pantry, or soup kitchen if you enjoy helping people in need.

Doing these things will only help your situation, I promise. When money is tight—as it will be for all of us from time to time—take advantage of free classes. The endless world on the internet and social media offers countless free learning opportunities. You will never regret taking time to mend yourself or volunteering your time.

God's Plan v. Layla's Plan

Exercise, healthy food, and lengthy talks with God seemed to be a better fit for me in terms of therapies. And, of course, the therapy I benefited from the most: cleaning. I was unstoppable when armed with bleach and a can of Lysol. I was obsessed with germs since Abi first came home from the hospital and wore the labels of "germaphobe" and "clean freak" proudly! Still, reflecting upon my situation at that time, I realize I was never actually happy—I was just in a perpetual state of fight or flight.

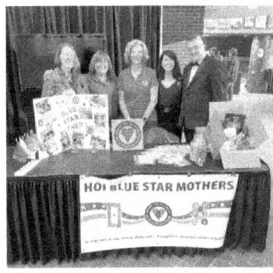 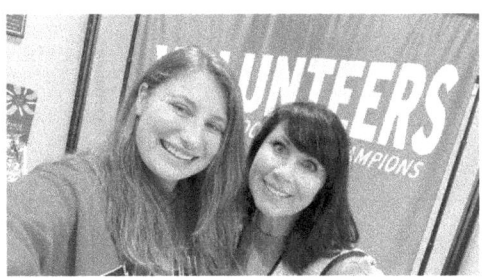

Although I prayed, participated in numerous Christ-centered activities, and was surrounded by friends who seemed to have my best interests at heart, I sometimes spent too much time indulging in my own pity parties. God was helping me grow from a self-centered child into a mature believer, but it would take time, and it would be painful. I would spend the next several years searching for the self that I had lost in the accident and discovering a new person within, who I never knew before.

I thought I had everything planned out in life, but none of this was in my crystal ball. Thankfully, my plan was no match for God's plan. God's plan differed from mine in numerous ways, and while much of that plan resulted in bliss, phases of it involved a great deal of agony. My plan did not involve getting married, but God blessed me with a husband straight out of a storybook. I did not intend on bearing or raising children, but God obviously had different plans in that area as well.

Another difference: instead of being a 30-year-old woman with a fancy career and a fat bank account, I was now a mother of two who worked countless dead-end jobs to help create financial stability for our family. One side effect of having only part-time jobs and being self-employed was that we were unable to carry group health insurance. This was not a big deal for someone who was healthy, but at the time, individual policies were not an option if you had a child whose medical records took up every square inch of a two-drawer filing cabinet.

My Christian perspective

By the time I became pregnant with Abigail, I was a Christian; I had accepted Christ when Noah was just over one year old. I was a bit wiser and older, had matured slightly, and was far less selfish than I had been when I became pregnant with Noah. In God's eyes, I still had a long way to go, though, so at the time, I believed that on October 17, 2002, He allowed havoc in my life to help me grow in my faith. I was hardheaded and set in my ways with a closed mind; how else would I become the person that God knew I could be?

Before you judge me for believing this, I want to explain myself. I was a new Christian who had never experienced a life-changing event of any kind, other than those of a positive nature. Growth and maturity can certainly come from tough times—in fact it usually does, like a "crucible moment." You are familiar with the phrase "no pain, no gain," right? When Lou Ferrigno morphs painfully from his human form into the Incredible Hulk, transforming from a non-believer into a mature Christian can be a painful process. When life is going well, you are not always growing the way that you do when times are difficult. I think about it in terms of the human body: you see results when you are disciplined enough to avoid the foods that pack on the pounds and can follow a strict cardio and weight-training routine. It is not always fun to be disciplined, but the results are always worth the sacrifices made.

Life as a Christian is very much the same. God knows that when you have no worries and when life is treating you well, you can become stagnant, even slothful. You become less and less dependent upon Him for money when the paychecks keep coming, and you no longer depend upon God to provide because you take for granted that the money will always be there. Likewise, when you and your loved ones are healthy and vibrant, you might become less inclined to go to Him each day in prayer about good health, and a distance can be created. Your relationship with God becomes shallow and one sided and He is very much aware when this occurs. In fact, He expects it. So one thing you can count on is that you will experience pain and discomfort from time to time and when you do, know that He is only helping you grow into the Christian that He knows you can become. There are a number of chapters in the Bible where we learn this, but if you are interested in reading a few, look for the following:

Hebrews 5:8

Psalm 119:71

1 Peter 5: 10

Acts 14:22

Psalm 119:67

Hebrews 12: 5-13

2 Corinthians 4: 16-18

Deuteronomy 8: 2-3

As I was discovering my newfound self and growing in my relationship with God, the four of us were plugging away at life in the general sense. We would find at times that we were on cruise control, while at other times we would be spinning recklessly out of control at the wheel. No matter what gear we were cruising along in, I put my faith in God and gave Him total control. I learned how to deal more constructively with the uphill battles, and slowly felt more at ease with my situation as I trusted that He would always care for us.

Understanding how God's plans differed from those that I had created at such an early stage in life may help you better grasp the pain of the predicament I felt I was in. It seemed to me that time and time again, I was knocked down for reasons I didn't understand. I was selfish, like most of us are when we are young, but God has shown me over the years that His plan was much more fulfilling than mine could have ever been. Now that I am married with children, I cannot fathom the idea of life without them. They have become the reason behind everything I do.

A Sense of Normalcy

Life seemed more "normal" for the time being, and we were even able to take a few family trips once Abi's appointments were scaled back. Her very first trip to California was in January 2005. We were able to introduce her to Brian's maternal family. We spent time with his mom, Sharon, and with our partners in crime, Doug, Tammy, and their girls. The feelings were of pure joy as this was technically our first family trip by plane. Abi did well on the plane rides and thoroughly enjoyed spending time with her new buddies—cousins Megan, Chandler, and Alyssa.

Spring came along and before we knew it, summer was

upon us. Noah turned five that summer and he would soon become a kindergartner. Besides routine appointments with Abi's pediatrician, pediatric ophthalmologist, neurosurgeon, and chiropractor, there was a period when we seemed to be out of the woods in terms of Abi's health. In August, Noah started school and settled into a new routine of full days instead of half-days like in pre-school. He embraced kindergarten with enthusiasm and nervous anticipation and fit right in with his new classmates.

October arrived, as did Abi's third birthday. The previous three years held many trials and celebrations, and the future looked bright. She had progressed in many ways, but we were smart enough to know that there would be huge mountains to climb at times and we were prepared—or at least we thought we were. If nothing else, we were armed with information and knowledge of what might become of Abi's conditions and care. I remained diligent in my crusade against what could be and often challenged God to show me miracles.

We knew there was always a risk of infection or malfunction of the shunt, and that Abi's best defense would be to keep illness out of her body at all costs. We were also prepared for the day that would inevitably come when she would need a shunt revision, during which the cord that coiled in her abdominal area would be extended. Since she was only the size of a fisherman's best catch at the time of the shunt placement, the cord would become shorter as she grew until it eventually needed to be replaced with a longer one. We figured if that were to become necessary, it would be well into the future, so felt safe shelving that worry for now.

What we did not anticipate, however, was the information that we learned after a trip to Omaha to see her original neurosurgeon. Since he was the doctor who had placed the shunt, we thought it would be best to keep him in the loop, and we trusted his abilities above all others. On November 27, 2005, we loaded up the family and necessary belongings to make our appointment the following day. It was a routine follow-up appointment where the neurosurgeon would perform some non-intrusive tests and check Abi to record her progress, but we could never have prepared ourselves for what we would find.

New Diagnoses

After the routine tests were performed, Brian and I had a chance to discuss our concerns, shedding light on the clumsiness that still had not improved like we had hoped. The doctor shared the same concerns about the imbalance between her left and right sides, and ordered an MRI that would be performed once we returned to Peoria, feeling there would be no harm in following up with her new neurosurgeon. He also felt a need for further neuropsychological testing and evaluations. We were introduced to yet another specialist, a neuropsychologist in Chicago.

Before we left Omaha, Abi's neurosurgeon informed us that, due to the brain injuries that Abigail had suffered, she would likely face learning disabilities and developmental complications. This was the first time that we participated in discussions about epilepsy or seizure disorder. We had wondered if the staring spells that she experienced in the past were, in fact, tiny seizures, but there was never any conclusive evidence, making it something that just fell by the wayside. Whatever the case may have been, we would have a clearer understanding after the MRI was performed.

Over the next two months, we were forced to sit on our hands and wait for the day of the MRI. Naturally, our imaginations got the best of us at times as we struggled to put this new information into perspective. Since Abi had only recently turned three, we had no reason yet to believe that learning disabilities would be another label to attach to her. We had already experienced developmental delays, but they did not seem outwardly noticeable in most instances. Because Noah was such a bright child with an amazing mind and imagination, we assumed that Abi would eventually show the same traits.

On January 31, 2006, Abigail underwent the highly

anticipated brain scan in Peoria at Children's Hospital, a place we had come to know all too well. The scan showed evidence of what the medical society termed "right frontal parietal hemisphere white matter loss" (loss of brain tissue in the right frontal part of the brain) as well as "cystic encephalomalacia" (softening of the brain due to degenerative changes in the nervous tissue) and "gliosis with hemosiderin deposit" (excessive development of supporting tissue intermingled with essential elements of nervous tissue). Enormous words for such a tiny girl, but what we would later learn would translate into learning disabilities, short-term memory loss, disconnections in thought processing, and mood instability, just to name a few.

The year 2006 was already shaping up to be one for the memory bank and it would progress into a whirlwind later. Hearing the findings of the MRI, we were referred to the University of Illinois at Chicago where we began a valuable relationship with a renowned pediatric neuropsychologist. Until then, I wasn't even aware that such a specialty existed, which made me both intrigued and anxious simultaneously. It was also here where we would finally see what Abi's brain injuries meant in terms of possible learning disabilities.

Another Sub-Specialist

We headed to Chicago after packing our bags and stuffing the car to the gills on March 7. Since our appointment was early in the morning the following day, we stayed in a hotel downtown to be well-rested and prepared for what was ahead of us. The pediatric neuropsychologist and her team put Abi through hours of testing as part of their March 8 evaluation, and she was a trooper. Any adult would have been completely exhausted and ready to throw in the towel after such rigorous physical and emotional tests, but my little miracle baby breezed right through it. Thankfully, she cooperated with all the expectations that were placed upon her, and in no time, we would have results to shed light on the severity of her brain damage.

Weeks later, we braced ourselves for the news that was packed into the long report of the team's findings. Since it was first brought to our attention that Abi had suffered several brain injuries, we expected that there would be some residual effects, but we did not know the extent of those effects. The reports from the testing by her neuropsychologist enabled her team to draw both short-term and long-term prognoses.

They found deficits that were consistent with what they called the "early neurologic insult" specific to hydrocephalus, prematurity, and skull fractures. This meant that we would anticipate "increased executive dysfunction," especially considering that as she grew older and more demand was placed upon her in classroom and social settings, she would not have all the skills necessary to respond to "increasing cognitive and behavioral demands" of her environment. They also noted that the left-sided weakness was consistent with the effects of the right parietal skull fracture that she suffered and that this could result in a significant risk for attention deficit disorder, learning difficulties, and social difficulties due to impulsive behavior. These difficulties would impact her ability to adapt daily in even minor situations that were outside of her normal day-to-day routines. As her school curriculum became more difficult and complex, the idea of her performing at or above grade level would be less realistic. We would find out year after year that these predictions could not have been any more accurate.

After getting all this news, we were even more cautious with our optimism about our little girl's future. At the time, it was difficult for us to process and apply to her current situation because she was not yet in school, but I noticed in my daily interactions with her that she was quite different from Noah at that age. I had already noticed problems with identifying colors, numbers, and letters, as well as what appeared to be difficulties with memorization and attention span. All I could do at that point was hold on tight for the bumpy ride and do all that I knew to do to prepare her, and the rest of us, for what lay ahead.

I had been in discussion with many different specialists on Abi's team of medical professionals and decided to take her to a physical rehabilitative medical specialist for evaluation. Five months later, our family embarked on another trip to Chicago, this time to see a new specialist who could shed light on Abi's physical needs, deficits, and prognoses. After a long meeting, question-and-answer session, and testing, we were able to get a confirmed diagnosis of cerebral palsy with a left-sided weakness and recommendations for how best to negate the effects. The doctor issued several recommendations for activities such as physical, occupational, and speech therapies; treatments, exercises, and stretches to improve the left-sided spasticity in her arm and leg; and a brace to immobilize her left elbow.

Riding Her Bike and Other Sports

The brace was meant to assist her in learning to ride her bike. Because of the left-sided weakness in her arm and leg, paired with the spasticity in the two appendages, she was unable to successfully ride her bike. She did not have enough strength in the left arm to hold it straight, causing the handlebars to inevitably turn the front wheel to the left as she pedaled. It was frustrating for her, as well as for me, as I watched her go around in circles on the bike when she did her absolute best to drive it in a straight line. It only took a couple of tries for her to completely give up on riding a training bike and it would be years before she would give it a go again.

The doctor also recommended that Abi not participate in most sports, especially those that involved any sort of bodily contact such as soccer, tumbling, and basketball. Since she was already involved in tap dance, that was allowable for the time being, and she would, through the next few years, progress to ballet and jazz. Among the rest of the recommendations that came from this particular visit were evaluations for nocturnal incontinence (which was thought to be the reason for the nighttime bed-wetting); individual therapy for her mood swings and family therapy to sort through the feelings that we were all experiencing; close supervision during all physical activities, especially swimming; further intermittent neuropsychological testing; and evaluation by a neurologist for staring spells that may have been minor seizures.

Our First EEG

We were absolutely overwhelmed with the information from the neuropsychologist and physical rehab specialist. We knew that our next step would be to take all this information back to her pediatrician and discuss the option of seeing a neurologist for evaluation. After speaking with the pediatrician, it was decided that we would proceed by first getting an electroencephalogram (EEG) reading on Abi's brain waves.

On September 6, Abi and I prepared for the next day's sleep-deprived EEG by staying up until midnight and waking at 4:00 a.m., according to the doctor's orders. This is not an easy task, especially when it involves a three-year-old. To pass the time, she and I played games and otherwise occupied ourselves until it was time to sleepily travel to our friendly local Children's Hospital.

We arrived an hour before the test to give the technician time to place all the necessary electrodes on her head and chest. These electrodes, held to her hair and skin with a paste-like adhesive, would monitor all the activity that occurred inside her tiny brain, and we would know for sure if the staring spells she was experiencing were, in fact, seizures. Once the preparation was finished, the technician quickly and kindly talked me through the details of the test and how it would progress. Then the lights were dimmed, and the tests began. Just as I dozed off at Abi's bedside, in came a team of medical personnel, one of which was a neurologist. This seemed a bit odd to me since it was not mentioned as part of the process, so I sat up attentively and was immediately thrown into a new world of wonder.

Learning About Seizure Medications

Soon after the EEG tests began, it was apparent to the medical staff that Abi was experiencing constant "misfires" in her brain waves, indicating seizure activity. Upon this explanation from the neurologist, my little one was admitted to the hospital for what he called complex partial seizure disorder. Since this was my first experience with such a term, I was like a deer in headlights as one medical professional after another came in and out of her hospital room, each throwing medical terms around as if it were no big deal. They immediately placed an IV in her arm, through which she was administered an anti-seizure medication called Phenobarbital.

Over the next two days, my sweet little baby girl was heavily sedated while the professionals monitored her brain activity and its response to the devilish drug. From that point forward, we would only have a foggy memory of who the non-medicated Abigail was. As it turned out, Phenobarbital would only be the first of a gamut of anti-seizure meds that Abi would take as her medical team played a game of trial and error to find the lesser of all the personality-changing drugs.

Complex Partial Seizure Disorder (focal seizures) according to Johns Hopkins:

Focal seizures can start in one part of the brain and spread to other areas, causing symptoms that are mild or severe, depending on how much of the brain becomes involved.

At first, the person may notice minor symptoms, which are referred to as an aura. The person may have altered feelings or sense that something is about to happen (premonition). Some people experiencing an aura describe a rising sensation in the stomach like riding on a roller coaster.

As the seizure spreads across the brain, more symptoms appear. If the abnormal electrical activity involves a large area of the brain, the person may feel confused or dazed, or experience minor shaking, muscle stiffening, or fumbling or chewing motions. Focal seizures that cause altered awareness are called focal unaware seizures or complex partial seizures.

The electrical activity of the seizure can remain in one sensory or motor area of the brain, resulting in a focal aware seizure (also called simple partial seizure). The person is aware of what is happening and may notice unusual sensations and movements.

After we returned home from our hospital stay, we were rudely awakened to the reality of a heavily medicated three-year-old. Now that she was a new preschool student, I had quite a lot of explaining to do to her teacher, principal, and administration. She missed a significant amount of school because she was too drugged up to function properly, and when she was in the classroom, she couldn't possibly have a productive day. The sweet blonde-haired, blue-eyed girl stumbled about as a drunken sailor would, which was one of the negative side effects of Phenobarbital. She staggered and fell even more often than she had before the medication, and her sweet demeanor transformed into that of a militant. Combative and confused, she was irritable and moodier than ever. She would cry in an instant, yelling and flailing about (commonly referred to as "meltdowns" by her teacher and by us). Her fellow students were distracted and confused by her behavior, and the teacher grew frustrated due to her lack of understanding of Abigail's condition.

Seeing the way this medication was affecting Abigail and everyone around her, we had no choice but to request another appointment with her new neurologist. From that point, we began the process of switching from one medication to another until, years later, we would finally come up with the correct medicine and dosage. We also learned that school district offered certain therapies, such as physical and occupational therapies, along with an Individualized Education Plan (IEP) that would assist Abi in progressing both academically and socially. We felt encouraged by this new information and looked forward to learning more.

To learn more about the medical terms and topics discussed in this chapter, visit this link:

www.SavingAbigailGrace.com

CHAPTER TEN

PT, OT, CTs, EEGs, and IEPs: What the Heck Are These?

FOR YEARS WE TRIED TO prepare ourselves for the day that Abigail would begin school, knowing that it could quite possibly be as much of a challenge for us as it would be for her. Now that the medication issue was at the forefront, all we could do was take each day as it came and keep an open mind to learning new things as we plugged along.

As Abi began preschool and was exposed to a classroom setting for the first time at the age of four, we quickly found that her school experience would be much different from Noah's. She had medical diagnoses, learning disabilities, and social shortfalls that placed her in an "at-risk" category, and right away we were informed of a process called an Individualized Education Plan, or an IEP. The basic purpose of the IEP was to find concerns or areas of weakness to focus on to assist the student's success. Because Abigail had been diagnosed with infantile cerebral palsy, hydrocephalus with a VP shunt, and motor and speech delays, she was a candidate for evaluations by the experts at school.

One month after she began school, Brian and I met with a team of professionals who followed Abi regularly as the IEP process unfolded. This team included her classroom teacher, the director of special education, a speech and language pathologist, an occupational therapist, a physical therapist, a school psychologist, a school social worker, and the principal. Each member of the team had a special focus, and all evaluated Abigail for a variety of strengths and weaknesses to develop her IEP for the school year. It was quite an interesting process, and we gained an enormous amount of knowledge as well as respect for the school officials. These specialists would devise my "dream team", of sorts, for Abigail's entire pre-K through eighth grade academic career.

After each of the educational professionals performed their tests and evaluations on Abigail, they presented us with their findings, goals, and objectives by way of a 15-page report. It was both fascinating and overwhelming in the beginning, and as the team discussed Abi's shortcomings and goals for improvement, I could do nothing but sit at the table and cry. And you know what? It's normal! Don't think you're weak if it happens to you— it very well may. A worthwhile team of academic professionals will embrace you through this experience, trust me. With Noah, everything seemed easy. He had no shortcomings to speak of and was, by all rights, the most "normal" child a parent could ever hope for. He was picture-perfect in his appearance, mannerisms, intelligence, and demeanor. Noah never really needed any extra assistance besides an occasional push in the right direction when he became distracted. I could not have been more ill-prepared for this very different experience with Abi.

Once my emotions subsided, I became entrenched in the report and in the assistance that would come from the school and all its experts. I knew that, since all would go as God planned, I had nothing to worry about, right? At least that was the theory, but those who know me also know that I find great difficulty in releasing control to anybody, even God Himself. Human nature, mixed with a type-A personality, forced me to hang on to as much control as I possibly could, which only led me to great heartache on many occasions. I had to trust that the school, guided by God's hands, would be able to take care of the situation, but I also would have to watch over the process like a mama bear to keep it all in check. That's what we moms do—we advocate for our children to the best of our abilities.

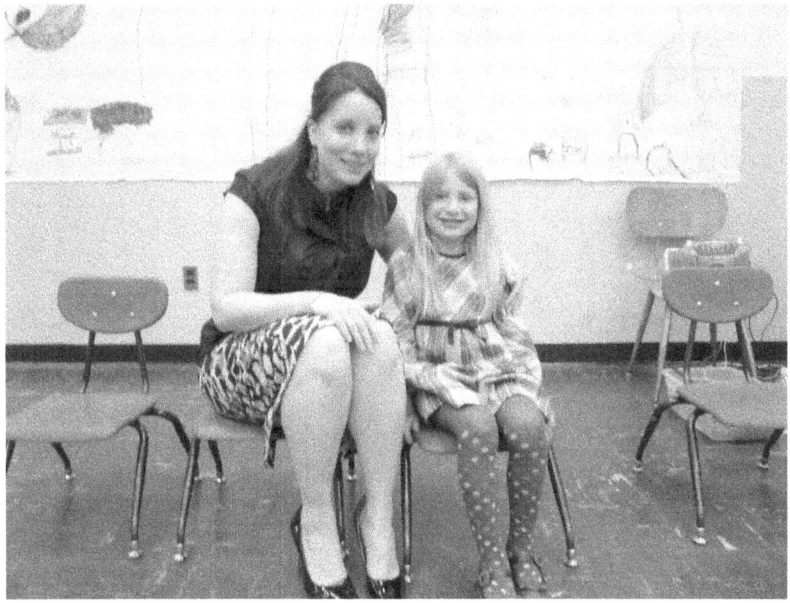

Abi with her Pre-K and first grade teacher

Understanding the IEP

The IEP was divided into two categories of assistance: educational services and environmental services. It was ultimately determined by Abi's team that she would receive speech and language therapy for 40 minutes a week, physical therapy for 30 minutes a week, and occupational therapy for 120 minutes a semester. She would also have extra homework from her speech pathologist for me to help her with at home, which delighted me.

The finding that was placed at the forefront of Abi's IEP was that she displayed a mild to moderate delay in language processing skills. This meant speech therapy was the largest part of her IEP, and she spent a great deal of time with her speech pathologist on activities aimed at improving her language processing skills. She would focus initially on determining items in a group that did not belong, identifying similar and different items, and providing attributes to given items. For example, upon identifying a sneaker, she could attribute it to running. Answering questions like who, what, when, where, and why would be the latter part of the objective.

Illinois Valley Central
Unit School District No. 321
Box 298
Chillicothe, IL 61523-
Ph: (309) 274-5418   Fax: (309) 274-5046

Speech and Language Evaluation Report
Confidential

Name: Abigail Slater

Date of Birth: 10/17/2002

Age: 4 Yrs 0 Mo

Sex F   Grade PreK

Language of child 000 English

Language of home 000 English

Ethnic Background

Date of Evaluation: 10/02/2006

Parent/Guardian Brian/Layla Slater

Address: 12139 N. Tall Trees

City: Dunlap, IL 61525-

Phone: (309) 278-5144

Attendance center Mossville School

Resident district: Illinois Valley Central #321

SPEECH AND LANGUAGE PROFILE:

Articulation:

Articulation is: ☑ Age Appropriate   ☐ Not Age Appropriate

Goldman Fristoe Test of Articulation - 2

The following sound errors were made during standardized testing: V, L, R, TH, NG.

Fluency:

Fluency is: ☑ Age Appropriate   ☐ Not Age Appropriate

Voice:

Voice quality is: ☑ Age Appropriate   ☐ Not Age Appropriate

Receptive Language:

Receptive language is: ☑ Age Appropriate   ☐ Not Age Appropriate

Peabody Picture Vocabulary Test III FormA

Testing established a standard score of 93, which falls within normal range (85-115) for Abigail's age.

Expressive Language:

Expressive language is: ☐ Age Appropriate   ☑ Not Age Appropriate

Expressive One-Word Picture Vocabulary Test

Testing established a standard score of 80, which falls slightly below the normal range (85-115) for Abigail's age. She appeared to have difficulty naming pictures. Many items she said she did not know. Other items, Abigail used general terms instead of a specific name (EX animal instead of answering duck).

Expressive Vocabulary Test

Testing established a standard score of 76, which falls below the normal range (85-115) for Abigail's age.

Oral Peripheral/Feeding/Swallowing:

Oral mechanism is: ☐ Adequate to support speech   ☐ Not adequate to support speech

Hearing Acuity: Hearing screening Date   by

☐ Pass   ☐ Fail   ☐ Could Not Test

☐ Wears hearing aid(s)/device.

☐ Student has prescribed hearing aid(s)/device, but does not wear it.

Auditory Discrimination:

Auditory discrimination abilities are   ☐ Age Appropriate   ☐ Not Age Appropriate

Medical History:

Page 1 of 2

Speech and Language Evaluation Report
Confidential

☐ No pathology noted on health record
☐ Noted pathologies from health record

Academic History:

School Year	Grade	Location	Special Programs

Summary:

☐ Articulation errors impact on student's ability to communicate.

☐ Articulation and language errors impact on student's ability to communicate

☑ Language deficits impact on student's ability to communicate.

☐ Dysfluencies impact on student's ability to communicate.

☐ Vocal abnormalities impact on student's ability to communicate.

☐ Communication abilities appear to be age appropriate.

Comments and Recommendations:

☑ Recommendations for speech/language services and placement will be determined at the IEP meeting.

Abigail displays age appropriate errors in articulation. Her fluency, voice, and receptive language skills appear to be age appropriate. Abigail displays a mild/moderate delay in expressive language skills.

Speech Language Pathologist

Angie Lagocki
Angie Lagocki, CCC-SLP

Additional copies to: **Attachments:**

Her left-sided weakness and lack of balance were reasons for the PT portion of the IEP, and her goal was to "progress gross motor skills to more fully participate in motor-based activities in the school setting." To achieve this, Abi performed a variety of exercises, such as running in a straight line and walking backward in a straight line for 8 to 10 feet at a time.

OT was only a small portion of the IEP but proved to be beneficial nonetheless. During her time with her occupational therapist, Abi worked on fine motor skills, such as learning to hold her writing utensils properly. She participated in finger exercises that helped her left hand become more functional and provided comfort for her right hand, which she used for writing and drawing.

A Sensory Diet

Where her environment was concerned, the plan allowed for certain exceptions in the classroom that provided comfort, such as sitting close to the teacher and the blackboard, as well as accommodations for her learning disabilities, such as displaying a daily paper schedule of classes on her desk. Because Abigail had a sensory processing disorder, part of her IEP included a "sensory diet." Her particular sensory issue was that she did not like to be touched by others (outside of our family), and she felt restricted by certain clothing, especially tights on her legs. She had anxiety about people being in her personal space, and would shut down when she felt threatened.

To address this, the sensory diet initially consisted of exercises with different textured items that she would become comfortable handling. For instance, she would feel a soft blanket on her cheek and describe it, or, in contrast, feel a rough surface on her cheek and describe it. These exercises would enable her over time to gain a level of comfort with being touched in appropriate ways.

As she grew older and graduated to kindergarten, the sensory diet evolved to include breaks from her work to create some mobility. Such breaks would consist of running errands for the teacher to the office, and handing out papers to her classmates to "help" her teacher. She gained a great deal of pride and acceptance when her teachers enabled her to perform small tasks that made her feel like she was contributing in an important way.

Also included in this "diet" were heavy work activities, seated activities, and oral motor activities. When she felt overwhelmed, Abi was encouraged to do wall push-ups or erase the chalkboards as part of the heavy work, and to perform "palm presses," where she would simply push her palms together, play with TheraPutty™, or squeeze a stress ball as seated activities. She was instructed to perform one of the sensory activities every 20 to 30 minutes for one minute throughout her school day to comply with her sensory therapy. All these activities helped alleviate her anxiety, giving her confidence and allowing her to channel some of her bottled-up energy in a positive way.

Each element of the IEP was revisited regularly with re-evaluations by the therapists and experts. To keep Brian and me informed of her progress, each member of the team also sent home regular reports indicating whether she was meeting goals that were set at the annual IEP meetings. As she progressed, some therapies were no longer required, bringing a new set of findings, reports, plans, and goals with each school year. The school was incredibly instrumental in Abi's social and academic progress. Her meltdowns slowly minimized over time. She had fewer crying spells and distracted her classmates less as medications were adjusted time and again.

What is a sensory processing disorder (SPD)?

According to *ADDitude Magazine*, SPD is a neurological condition that interferes with the body's ability to receive messages from the senses and convert those messages into appropriate motor and behavioral responses.

It inhibits a person's ability to filter out unimportant sensory information, like the background noise in a bustling café, making them feel overwhelmed and overstimulated in certain environments.

SPD also interferes with the body's ability to process and act on information received by sight, sound, touch, smell, and taste.

Building Important Relationships— It Takes a Village

Our relationships with the faculty and staff at school were increasingly important and necessary, so I became a permanent fixture on campus by often volunteering in Noah's and Abi's classrooms. I later became a substitute teacher to earn a paycheck for the work I performed at the school, furthering my familiarity with its processes and strengthening my relationships there. I encourage all parents to become involved in their children's academic lives to strengthen bonds with the teachers and administration. This team effort has such a significant role in a child's growth.

Equally important are the relationships that we grow with our children's medical team. Abigail continued to see her neurologist every four weeks while we were closely monitoring her behavior, schoolwork, and medicine. We played a constant game of trial and error to find the delicate balance between medicine and its effects on her, while minimizing her risk of seizures. Some days were easier than others, but I was happy with her progress and the attention that she was getting from all who were involved in her care.

Through daily contact with Abi's teacher, I found that she was still running into objects in the classroom and falling more than occasionally. Because the medicine made her so drowsy, she had a difficult time boarding and getting off the bus, so the driver monitored her closely. Around this time, she became incontinent while she slept, giving us no choice but to put her back in Pull-Ups® at night. This was quite a blow, considering she had gone nearly a full year without a single wetting accident and had been fully potty-trained. We could tell it affected her negatively and made her incredibly self-conscious.

Getting the Medications Right for Abigail

After Abi had taken Phenobarbital for several months, the neurologist, Brian, and I decided the medication was doing more harm than good in terms of her emotions and physical abilities. Her neurologist then began weaning her off it and onto a second drug called Depakote. It did not take long to see that it also had a very negative effect on her, and her behavior became a major concern. If there was a side effect, Abi exhibited it. She was wobbly on her feet, sleepy, and complained of dizziness often. Once I shared these concerns with her neurologist, he decided to introduce a third medication in hopes that its effects would be less negative, while keeping the seizure activity at bay. She was weaned off Depakote and onto Tegretol, and we saw an improvement in her behavior, but the drowsiness caused by the drug made it impossible for her to stay awake. Within 15 minutes of taking it, she would be asleep for an hour or two. She absolutely could not function on Tegretol and was, once again, missing quite a lot of school.

By January 2007, Abigail was on her fourth anti-seizure medicine. This time, she took a drug called Keppra, which seemed to have the least negative side effects of the medicines we had tried up to this point. She was at least able to function and behave properly at school, but the bed-wetting issue seemed to get worse. After seeing one specialist after another in the urology field, we determined that there was no reason for the incontinence other than the fact that the medicine was causing her to sleep so deeply that she was unable to wake up to use the bathroom. All her organs had grown normally and were functioning properly, and her specialists assumed that she would eventually outgrow the problem, but it might not happen until she no longer needed to take anti-seizure medication.

Throughout the process of finding the medicine with the least number of side effects, Abigail was incredibly emotional. The poor little girl had no idea for most of the year who she was or what she was doing. She was completely out of it most of the time, and we began to wonder who the real Abigail was. We hadn't known the non-medicated version of Abi for very long, and we knew that the medicated version was so difficult to live with that I thought about running away from home every day. She cried about anything that did not go exactly the way she wanted, and the meltdowns both at school and at home were occurring more regularly with each change in medication. Raised voices, a dirty look, and even toys being out of place made her cry.

She never seemed to smile and almost nothing made her happy. This was absolutely heartbreaking for Brian and me to witness and quite trying for all of us.

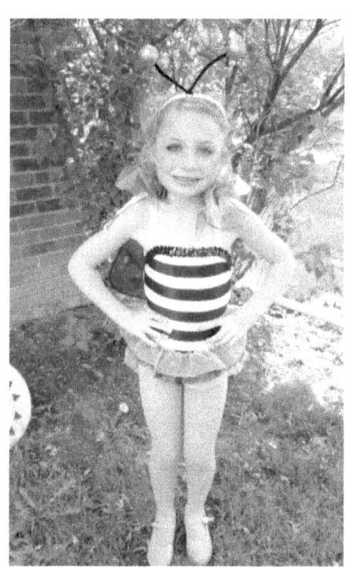

Abi dressed for one of her dance recitals

There were times when I arrived at her classroom to volunteer, and she made it so difficult for me to stay that her teacher asked me to keep my distance for a while. She would be in tears for much of the time that I was there and would completely freeze up while in my presence because she could not separate the "me" at home from the "me" at school. My presence meant that she no longer had to function like a student at school. In her mind, if I was there, she could behave as if she were at home and that obviously was not beneficial to her or to her classmates and teacher. This made my heart hurt because I felt isolated and as if I were a bad influence on her behavior.

Abigail became involved in dance class, which became more difficult while we were changing medication. She loved to tap dance, but there were times when all she wanted to do was sit on the floor and watch the other girls perform. She was always tired and lethargic, and when she refused to dance, I would be forced to take her home to not distract the others. I knew it was good for her to be involved in dance class nonetheless because of her physical disabilities. She eventually grew as a tap dancer and became a ballet and jazz dancer as well, but it only lasted a few years, fizzling out like most of her other extracurricular activities.

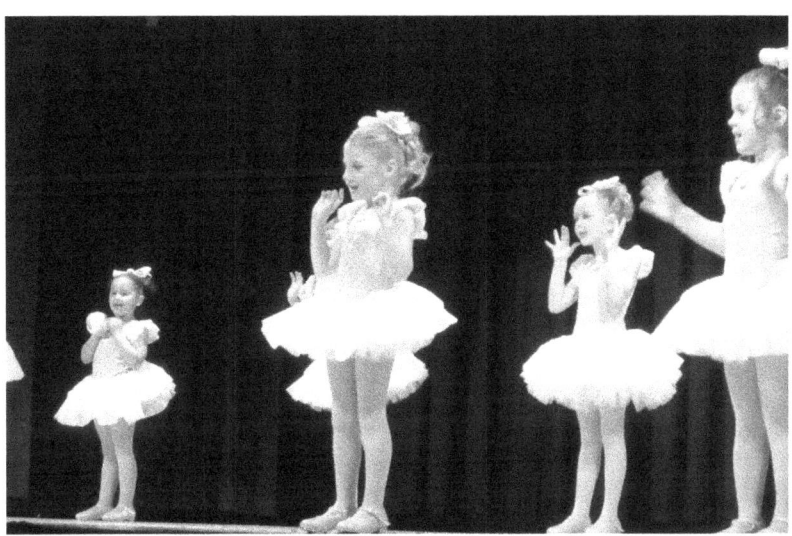

There are many different anti-epileptic medications available. Finding the right medication can be a long process of trial and error and it requires incredible patience. Because there is no one-size-fits-all approach to controlling epilepsy, approach this challenge knowing that it can be tedious and frustrating but once the right med is found, it will be worth it.

Noah's Progress

Meanwhile, all was going well with Noah and the other areas of our lives. Noah was involved in hockey, and it was a blast to watch him practice and compete. We thoroughly enjoyed watching our local hockey team play on the ice and made regular family outings of it. Noah and his team even got to play on the same ice as the Peoria Rivermen during a break one night, which was the highlight of his year! Seeing him develop a passion for it was exciting. He only played for a year before trying various other sports, such as basketball and baseball, which were also fun to watch and much less expensive than hockey.

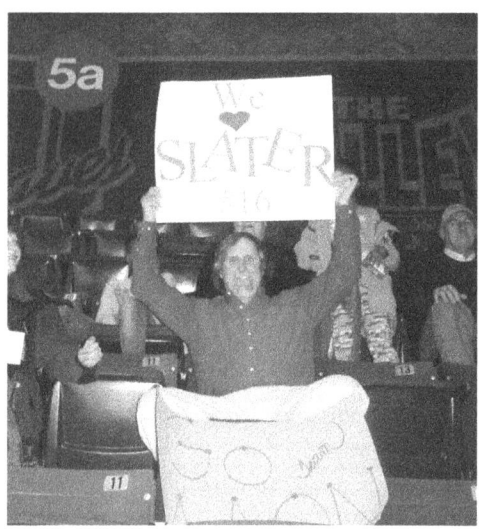
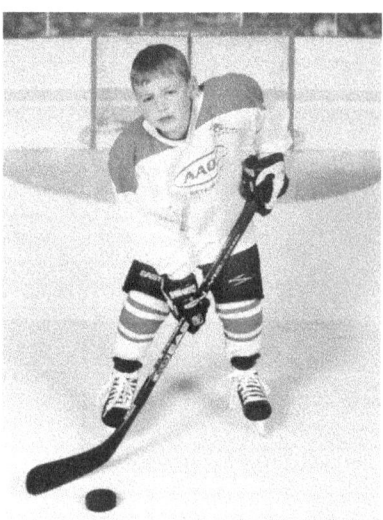

Sometimes You Lose It

We were still very much involved in church, and our church family had become very important to us, especially as we went through such trying times with Abi's medicine and poor behavior. There were times when I all but lost my religion on my way out the door to church because she frustrated me so much. I repeatedly had to tell myself that it was the medicine that was to blame for her behavior, but that didn't necessarily calm me down or make me feel less hopeless. Because I had to always be strong for Abi and the family, my mantras became "Suck it up, buttercup" and "Just keep swimming."

Tattooed on my memory is a specific time when I allowed

the medicine's effects to send me home from church in tears. It was a Sunday morning, the most stressful time of our week, and I had instructed Abi to get changed from her pajamas into her church clothes while I showered. Exiting the shower, I found that she was still standing where I left her, in her pajamas. Already running late, I now had to get her dressed and do her hair all while she was complaining and crying. I scolded her and told her how I wanted her to be more independent. My temper was getting the best of me, and I am quite certain that I threw around a few curse words. By the time we left for church, I was both furious and disgusted with myself for losing my cool.

Once we were in church, Abi began her usual routine of crying over perceivably nothing, and I snapped. She had a habit of taking the seat of whoever got out of their chair because she thought it was funny. This time it was the pastor's son who fell victim to her silly game. He was upset with her, they began to fight over the chair, and she had a major meltdown. Not being able to stand a second more of her antics, I drove home by myself and cried all the way there. Once home, I called my mom and cried through the entire church service. When Brian called me for a ride home (I had left him and the children carless), I could not bear the thought of getting out of the car to find them. I was embarrassed by my behavior and Abi's and never wanted to show my face to the congregation again. Those sorts of things happened often enough, and although I tried to remain calm and understanding, I could not help but react negatively at times. Afterward, I would feel depressed, self-pitying, and hopeless for any sense of normalcy.

During this time, Brian and I decided to join a gym because I needed a consistent way to burn off steam and calories while producing endorphins that would change my attitude. Abi and Noah enjoyed playing with the other children in the gym's childcare class, and Abi seemed to get along well with them. Eventually, gym time became a natural part of our family routine, and it served us all well. Self-care was an important aspect to explore as the parent of a child with disabilities. Intentionally carving out time for myself each day was essential to both my and Abi's wellness. A strong, mentally and physically healthy parent is best equipped to support their family throughout such a stressful time.

Another part of my routine was taking Abi to the hospital every four to six weeks to get blood work done. Because the medicines she took could have adverse effects on her internal organs, her neurologist made sure that we had trough levels performed regularly to confirm the medication levels in her blood were adequate. At first this was difficult for her and, in turn, made it difficult for me. She cried and reached a point where she wouldn't get in the car if I told her what we were doing or where we were going. As time passed, though, she accepted it for what it was and even assisted the nurse in getting the blood samples. She became quite a helpful little pin cushion! It was amazing what a few stickers from the nurses could do for a little one's compliance.

After discussing with Abi's neuropsychologist all the behavioral issues we were dealing with, Brian and I, at her recommendation, decided it was a good idea to get a second opinion. The neuropsychologist had a renowned colleague at the Cleveland Clinic, noted as one of the best pediatric neurology clinical researchers. Upon her recommendation in May of 2007, my dad and I packed Abi into my Pontiac Aztek and drove to Cleveland.

Our Adventures in Cleveland

Brian stayed behind to work and to take care of Noah since Abi, Dad, and I planned to be gone for nearly an entire week. Abigail was admitted to the hospital for a minimum of three days while the pediatric neurology team performed a continuous EEG on her brain waves. The hope was to determine exactly how often she was having seizures over the extended period and to pinpoint the part of the brain where the "misfires" began.

Up to this point, Abi's seizure disorder had been quite a

mystery to her neurologist in Peoria. The original EEG revealed an almost constant state of misfires in all areas of her brain, making it difficult to pinpoint the exact location responsible for the occurrences. Her EEG readout showed massive scribbles (called spikes) large enough to immediately concern her specialists. All they knew to do at the time was pump her full of drugs and watch closely to observe the outcome. For Brian and me, that was not an acceptable answer, and while she was on one medication after another, I was calling every specialist I knew to find a more permanent course of action. And so, we ended up at Cleveland Clinic with the best possible team we could have in our corner to find real answers. For the first time in what seemed like forever, I had hope.

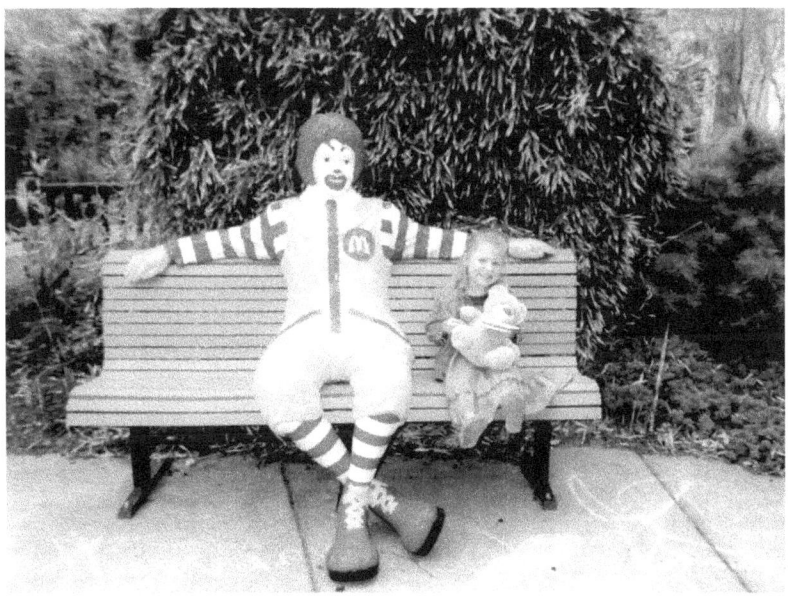

Abi at the Cleveland Ronald McDonald House before her EEG

Our first stop once we reached the city was Ronald McDonald House. This was the place where Dad and I laid our heads when we were not at Abi's bedside. I felt like a pro when we checked into the facility and were led to our room because of my experience with Rainbow House in Omaha. With colorful decor and pleasant fragrances, it was a homey facility that housed up to 74 guests at a time and was equipped with plenty of amenities. There was a fully-equipped kitchen where there was almost always a meal of some sort provided, as well as a library, laundry facilities, and a family resource center. The grounds were heavily secured with gates, ensuring that all guests could feel safe and surrounded by friendly faces and beautiful scenery. We were fortunate to have such an affordable housing option while focusing on my little girl, who stayed just a hop, skip, and a jump away in a hospital bed.

After checking in and unloading all our belongings into our new resting place, Dad, Abi, and I made our way to dinner, giving us time to enjoy ourselves before taking Abi to the clinic. My dad was always good for a ton of laughs and had such a carefree spirit, so we thoroughly enjoyed ourselves as we prepared for what the next three days would hold. Abi, of course, had not a care in the world and was extremely excited to get the chance to sit next to a faux Ronald McDonald when Dad and I were getting settled at the house. She wanted to talk only about Ronald and her teddy bear, to which she always clung tightly. Her innocence was both comforting and heartbreaking to me because I knew the next day would be an unpleasant one for all of us.

Abi's Big Neurology Day

The next morning, we rose early and boarded the shuttle that Dad and I would become familiar with during our stay. We would soon be eyeball-deep in paste, electrodes, monitors, and medical staff, but all the discomfort would hopefully bring about highly anticipated answers. There were a multitude of questions we hoped to get answers to: Why was she having seizures? What area(s) of her brain were responsible for the activity? Is medicating her condition the only option? Is the medicine causing more harm than good? Where do we go from here?

Once Abigail was admitted to the clinic, we were visited by the director of the Neurology Center at the main campus. She would be the lead doctor overseeing the tests and presenting results in layman's terms, ultimately leading to a plan for Abi's future. With a tiny frame and a firm handshake, she was a force to be reckoned with, commanding the room with her presence. I liked her right away, and my dad and I were immediately confident as she explained the entire process to us and what they would be looking for. Suddenly, I was at ease.

Our team of neurologists and nurses was vast and knowledgeable. They made the situation comfortable for Abi, as well as for my dad and me, by keeping food in our bellies and drinks in our hands. Someone was always asking if we needed anything, which helped keep our minds free of worry and unnecessary burdens. Like most of the experiences we had at various hospitals in the past, there was something soothing and comforting about being surrounded by the sterile smell, buzzing machinery, and medical staff fluttering about at all hours.

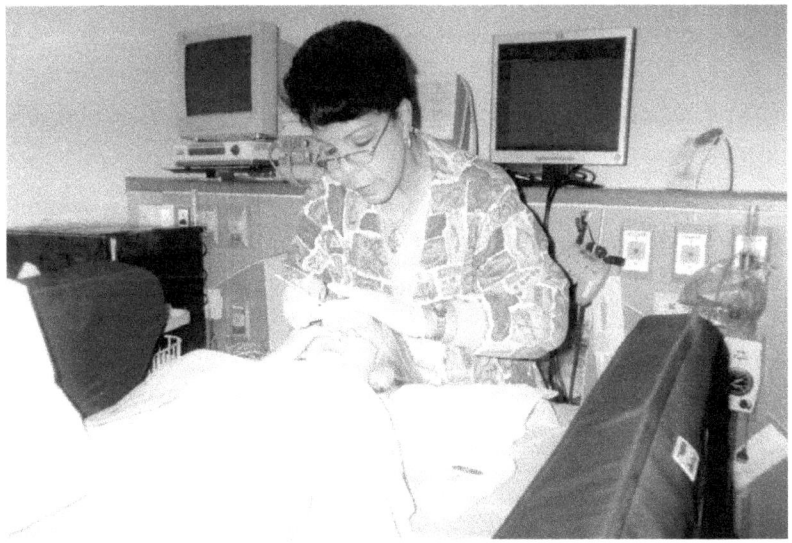

Abi's EEG technician applying the electrodes

Before too long, we were introduced to a brown-haired EEG technician with mocha skin and a beautiful, bright white smile, who was the one hooking Abi up to all the electrodes needed to perform the test. She had endless energy and such a positive spirit that we could not help but to immediately fall head over heels for her. She talked to Abi through the entire process, making sure she always knew what was coming next, all the while joking and laughing with us. My dad even brought out his signature cackle several times during her visit, which made us laugh that much harder.

With the mood light and the three of us at ease, the technician began scrubbing the oils off each site that would house an electrode, making it stick to Abi's scalp. This was done with what looked like an oversized Q-Tip, so the technician had a fun time providing light-hearted commentary about that. Next, she applied a paste to each spot and then placed the electrodes on the globs of paste. I cannot recall the exact number of electrodes that were placed throughout my daughter's long, thick mane of blonde hair, but it was near 50. After she was finished with the application, she moved onto Abi's chest and repeated the process, this time with less than 10 electrodes.

Each of the tiny metal buttons led to a common box with thin wires of several different colors. This box was plugged into a monitor where all brain activity would be recorded for later analysis by the team. Abi was also adorned with leads that monitored her heart rate, breathing patterns, oxygen levels, and other vital signs at all times for the next three days. A video camera recorded all her outward activity, allowing the team to compare her brain's activity with what they saw occurring externally. For instance, they would be able to see if Abi's body made certain movements when her brain waves spiked on the EEG readout.

What a scene this was once all preparation was complete! Here lay a tiny, four-and-a-half-year-old girl full of infinite energy, whose only job was to lay in one spot for the next 72 hours. Keeping her entertained was an exhausting chore, but I had the best entertainment of all with me: the man who happened to be the light of both of our lives (outside of Brian and Noah, that is)—Abi's grandpa and my sweet dad. He would stop at nothing to make sure his granddaughter was well-equipped for what was, at times, a bumpy ride. We had coloring books, crayons, movies, video games, board games, books, and Abi's bedside landline to occupy our time. Grandpa even brought out his card tricks and taught both of us some new card games.

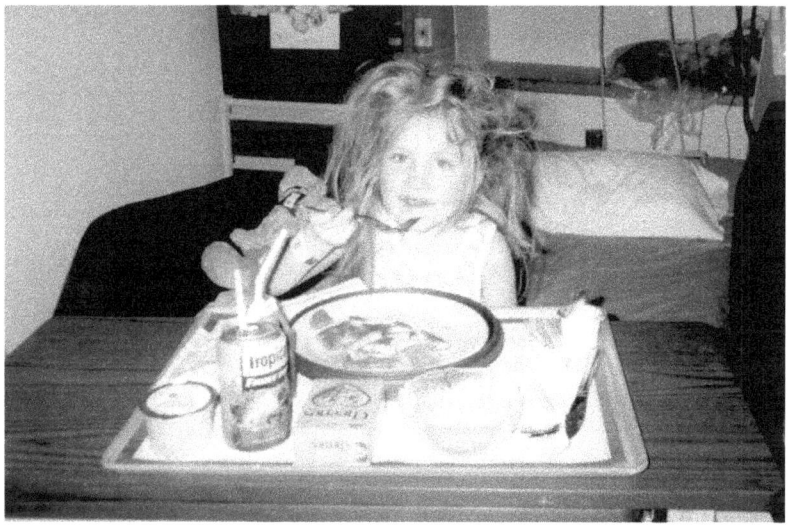

Over the next few days, Dad and I took turns going back to Ronald McDonald House via shuttle only when we needed showers or when Dad needed to sleep at night. Abi was never left in her research bed alone; I hated the thought of her being scared in such a big, unfamiliar place filled with strangers in white coats. I spent each night in her room with her, giving me the opportunity to keep a close watch over her every move.

There were even nights that I slept on her bed at her feet just to be near her. I could often feel her tossing about in the night with what seemed like tremors or quick convulsions, but the staff assured me that they were not seizures. Still, I was unable to catch a decent night's sleep during our stay because I was on pins and needles at the thought that the team might find something we weren't prepared to learn.

Like Santa Claus appearing before an adoring child, Dad would come back to the clinic early in the mornings with two cups of steaming, fragrant coffee in hand—one for me, of course. He had always been my favorite coffee companion, even dating back to the NICU days in Omaha when we would begin each morning at Starbucks. Each time he reappeared, Abi and I had new light in our faces and spring in our steps; he always seemed to bring sunshine into the room, even on the darkest days. The calmness I felt in my soul during this time together will forever be stamped on my heart like a Sharpie on paper.

Although Abi was much more comfortable lounging than most other preschoolers, she had her moments while shackled to her bed. When she had to potty, it took a team of us to get her to the toilet with all the wires and the black box to which they were attached. But we made a game of it, joking about her jungle hair, calling her a wild child, and growling like a lion to add some humor. She made lots of calls to her daddy and brother to tell them all about her time in the small room with an even smaller bed. It was a very long three days, but once it was all over, we were thankful that we had made that long trek to Cleveland Clinic, and I was grateful Dad made it with me. I have never been a fan of traveling distances on my own, and his company was a blessing I will always treasure. I truly do not know what I would have done without my dad during this time.

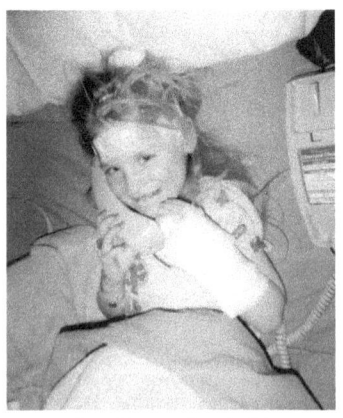

Abi talking to her daddy on the phone

Our Test Results

The neurology team found that, while there was obvious evidence of misfires, the chance of Abi experiencing full-blown seizures was so small that they saw no need to take the risk of medicating her. We were given the option to wean her off her meds completely, while monitoring her closely for future evidence of seizure activity. This news made me ecstatic, and I happily made the decision to kick the medicine to the curb, at least for the time being.

With this good news at the forefront of our minds, we ventured back to Ronald McDonald House one last time and gathered our belongings for the trip home. While I was at the clinic with Abi, Dad had already laundered all the bedding and cleaned our room in preparation for check out. We paid our bill and thanked the excellent staff before exiting the iron gates of the property. There was just one last thing to do before we left the impressive city of Cleveland.

A Few Moments of Joy

Dad had always been an admirer of French impressionist Claude Monet's artwork and had read in the newspaper that his *Monet in Normandy* original pieces were on display at the Cleveland Art Institute, so we decided to take a peek. It was a lasting memory for me to see my dad enjoy himself thoroughly after being cooped up in a hospital room for days. Watching him was like watching a child discover Disneyland for the first time: innocent and awe-inspiring. It was the true fulfillment of a dream for him, and he exuded pure joy, which filled Abi and me with utter delight.

After taking our time strolling through the Monet exhibit, we cruised through downtown Cleveland and Dad experienced yet another first. Although he had traveled to many cities in the United States while in the Army, he had never seen Lake Erie, and since it was only a couple of blocks from where we were, he wanted to drive to its shores. So, with Abi content in the backseat, we drove alongside the shores of Lake Erie, taking in the beauty of the vast body of water and the cloudy, dark Cleveland day. With the fresh spring air feathering our faces and my dad's choice of music serenading us from the Aztek's speakers, it was a remarkable end to a trying but successful visit. We headed home fulfilled, satisfied, and cautiously excited about our new findings and what it might mean for Abi's quality of life.

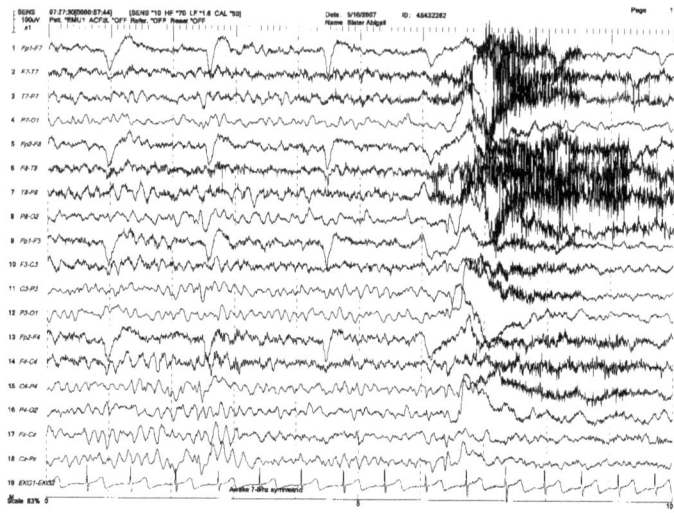

We arrived home from Cleveland in time for the school year to end and for summer to begin. Now that Abi would be free of medication, we would have the summer to adjust and monitor her for signs of seizures or any unusual behavior. It would be interesting to see how she would be affected by the absence of meds. We hoped to see a total shift in her behavior, as well as improvement with the incontinence while she slept. It was still early enough in her school career that I was optimistic about her studies and grades.

To learn more about the medical terms and topics discussed in this chapter, visit this link:

www.SavingAbigailGrace.com

CHAPTER ELEVEN

School Daze

THE SUMMER STARTED WITH A bang. Abi was still involved in dance and loving every minute of it. She became less timid on stage and made friends with the other tiny dancers. Noah joined a baseball team, which kept us busy in the heat but was worth it when we saw how much he enjoyed hitting the ball with all his might.

Abigail began OT through Children's Hospital as ordered by her physiatrist. A physiatrist specializes in physical medicine and rehabilitation, or PM&R. They treat, among other things, neurological disorders; in Abi's case, she was seen for her cerebral palsy. The orders also involved speech and physical therapy, but after evaluations for both, we were placed on a long waiting list for speech therapy, and it was found that PT was unnecessary at the time. So for the duration of the summer, she saw her OT once a week to work on fine motor skills such as those required in handwriting and grasping objects like pencils, crayons, and eating utensils. This would be the last of outpatient therapy services through the hospital, and further services would be provided by the school's experts.

Abi made it through the summer without any epileptic episodes and was still med-free, thankfully. She enjoyed her time being a typical little girl playing outside with the neighborhood kiddos and her big brother. She began her second year of preschool on August 30, 2007, with an updated IEP and some minor changes. Seemingly back on track after participating in OT over the summer, we never did get a call for an opening in speech therapy, so it was no surprise that the most demanding portion of the IEP for that school year would be focused on that.

She picked up where she left off the previous year, as most goals had not yet been met, but she was working hard to achieve enough to progress into kindergarten. Quarterly reports noted that she was improving in most areas in the classroom, especially where her social skills were concerned. The meltdowns were minimal, and she seemed to be making friends with her fellow classmates.

Her fine motor skills were progressing nicely, and she participated in activities such as stringing beads, playing with Play-Doh, and using drawing tools. She also worked to strengthen her gross motor skills by riding bikes with training wheels and scooters, as well as swinging on the playground swings—one of her favorite pastimes. Abigail had become quite good at expressing herself artistically and loved interacting in the dramatic play area at school by performing music, dancing, and drawing.

Since she had made such great strides in most categories at school, we now found ourselves on cruise control and could cautiously breathe a sigh of relief. She was well on her way to accomplishing all the goals that were set by each of her therapists as part of the IEP, and everyone involved in her care was proud of her hard work and focus.

My "Free" Time

With Abi and Noah advancing well, I found myself with some time on my hands. I had become more involved in the community, at church, and at school, and was able to focus my attention on helping others who were less fortunate. Since college, I had been passionate about volunteering and working within my community to improve situations for others, so I was now working as a tutor and mentor through a charity called Common Place in Peoria. After completing a training course and earning my certificate, I was assigned a woman who was an adult learner in the program. It was my mission to help her with reading, writing, math, and whatever else she needed help with at the time. We met on Tuesdays and Thursdays at the local library, where we went over the lessons I prepared ahead of time. My time with her was valuable, and we grew to like and appreciate each other very much.

The church was growing and finding that it could no longer function on the bare-bones volunteer pool that had previously been sufficient. I began to pick up the slack wherever I was needed. In addition to singing in the choir, singing special solo music, and assisting in the women's ministry, I was devoting more time to teaching various children's age groups. I subbed in junior church when needed, taught some Sunday school classes, and served in the nursery regularly. My soul was fed, and my heart was content while I was serving the Lord.

The school had just introduced a mentoring program, and I became a mentor to an underprivileged fourth-grade girl. Once a week, I met her in the teacher's lounge. There she could enjoy some time with an adult other than her teacher, in a safe environment where she would not be teased by her classmates and could take a much-needed break from the stresses of everyday life. I brought scrapbooking materials, and other days I would just read with her. She liked simple stories like those found in the *Skippyjon Jones* books, and I theatrically read that collection to her and took her mind off her troubles while she relaxed for half an hour at a time.

During that time, I served on the parent advisory board for preschool and attended monthly meetings with parent representatives from all the local school districts. It was during these meetings that we were informed of events in the district, as well as of any needs the district had in terms of funding and volunteers. This was a great way to be involved in the highest level of decision-making for the preschool that my daughter attended. I was able to offer my opinions and solve problems that directly related to our family, therefore feeling I had some control, albeit small, in my daughter's care.

Epilepsy In Our Home

We were blissfully plugging along and enjoying the simple things that life had to offer. This was a new concept for us since Abigail's arrival five years earlier, and we basked in it like a lizard in the sunshine. Abi was still wetting herself nightly, wearing pull-ups to bed, and struggling from time to time with school-related issues, but it was nothing that we could not handle. Considering all the warnings that had come to us from her various specialists since her birth, we felt lucky to see what progress had unfolded.

Then, what we had all braced ourselves for in the past happened. On the morning of May 3, 2008, we awoke to a choking noise unlike anything we had ever heard before. Earlier that morning, Abi had stumbled into Brian's and my bedroom around 7:00 a.m. She tried to wake Brian up but since it was a Saturday, he was reluctant to rise and instructed her to go back to bed. Somehow, Noah had ended up in bed with us the night before, and when we heard the odd noise about an hour and a half later, he, unfortunately, was the first to find its source. Noah entered the kitchen to find Abi lying flat on her back on the hard floor, totally dazed and unaware of her surroundings. Of course, this scared the daylight out of Big Brother, and he frantically called for us from the kitchen.

When Brian and I reached her, she was unable to respond to our voices and could not answer our questions. Dazed, her blue eyes were completely blank as she stared into the distance, unable to focus on our faces. She could not nod or shake her head to respond to us, nor did she seem to hear a word we said. What she was able to do, however, was touch Brian's face. As she lay on the floor in front of the oven, she reached up and felt her favorite guy's face, caressing it almost as a blind person would. Brian finally picked up her head and cradled it in his enormous hand and as he did, she began to heave as if to vomit. Alarmed, he scooped her up into his arms and ran at full speed to the bathroom, but she was unable to vomit.

Meanwhile, I called her pediatrician's after-hours line because I did not have a clue as to what was going on with her and I needed instruction on what to do next. The nurse on the other end of the line instructed me to take her to the emergency room immediately. We all frantically threw on our clothes and rushed out the door. I was terrified.

We arrived at the ER at Children's Hospital, and Abi was still in a daze, unable to comprehend what was occurring. She had not said a single word and appeared to be completely exhausted. At first, Brian and I wondered if she was experiencing a shunt malfunction, but after the medical personnel reviewed the CT scan and x-ray results, that possibility was thankfully ruled out. After we discussed all our findings and Abi's behaviors with the doctors at the ER, it was beginning to sound like what we were seeing were the aftereffects of a major seizure.

She was finally admitted to room G226 at Children's Hospital of Illinois at approximately 4:30 p.m. that day and would stay for the next three days. She finally said her first word about two and a half hours after we found her on the floor. When asked by an ER nurse what her name was, she responded in an almost non-existent voice, "Abi." For much of the day, she was in and out of consciousness and the blank stare on her face didn't really change until hours later. Now that she was admitted, she took it easy until her neurologist and neurosurgeon could see her the following day.

After someone has a seizure of any kind, they will typically experience total exhaustion. The level of exhaustion may depend on the severity and/or the type of seizure. It takes an incredible amount of energy, both physically and mentally, and it is important to let that person sleep it off. And, as long as they are safe from any potential environmental harm, it's best to let the seizure run its course while they are lying on their side, preferably with something soft under their head.

Thankfully, we had many visitors arrive to keep us company that first day, most of which were friends from church. An older couple with whom we had formed a bond over the years offered to take Noah for a while, which afforded him a nice time away from the hospital. What an incredible blessing that was! While they were away, they had lunch and went shopping for some games and toys for Abi and Noah, providing them with a positive outlet to put their energy the following day. Brian and Noah left the hospital around 10:30 p.m. that night so that Noah could try to get some rest before coming back the next morning, and I sleepily prepared my resting place in a recliner at Abi's bedside.

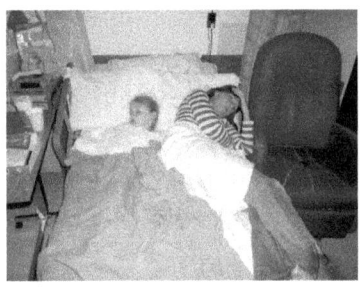

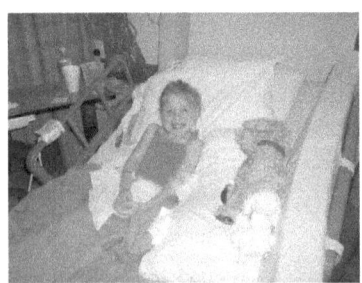

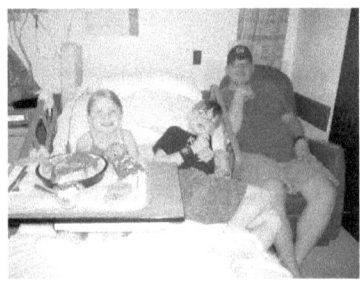

An Unexpected Moment of Friendship

Late that night, after everyone was snuggled tightly in bed, Abi received a roommate who had also been admitted upon suffering a seizure. I immediately recognized the blondie when her mother and nurse brought her into the room. Her name was Jade, and she had been a classmate of Abi's in developmental therapy three years prior. I remember being heartbroken when we first met her in class because she was heavily medicated, making her unable to walk without stumbling, and her speech was incredibly delayed. She was a beautiful girl whose presence was like a flashing neon light, reminding me of how blessed we really were to not have to deal with such calamity and frustration as she and her family did. (I often wonder how she is doing now that she is most certainly a young adult woman.)

That night, we were visited by my pastor, who stopped by unannounced to pray with and for us all. Word travels quickly in the church, and his visit was much-appreciated. After he left for the night, Jade's mother and I talked into the wee hours of the next morning. Our conversation, filled with a variety of emotions, was both informative and eye-opening, revealing the struggles her family had faced since Jade was born. Jade had suffered from a seizure disorder since she was an infant, and even with heavy doses of the most intrusive medications available, they were never able to control recurrences. Her quality of life was minimal, and there seemed little hope for improvement. In that room, otherwise devoid of emotion and color, I could feel the heaviness of her mind and body as the painful words were thrust from her mouth into the air, occupied with the lull of machines.

Parents, we must not only seek support from others, but we must pray to also be the support that others need. That particular night meant so much to both Jade's mother and me because neither of us had many others in our lives who could relate to what we were experiencing. I am convinced that God strategically placed our girls in the same hospital room simultaneously because He knew we needed each other. Please do not be afraid to open yourself up to these types of blessings as you navigate your own journey.

When we could no longer keep our eyes open, we both laid our heads to rest around 1:00 a.m., only to be forcefully awakened that morning by the doctors and nurses who discussed the plan to conduct another EEG the next morning. Because it was to be a sleep-deprived test, we would again have a late night and early morning, being allowed to sleep only from 1:00 a.m. to 5:00 a.m.

Playing the Waiting Game

Because this day would be one of waiting for the next day's procedure, we would spend an exorbitant amount of time playing games like Uno®, checkers, and dominoes, and passing the hours putting together puzzles, reading books, and drawing pictures. Some of our friends from church came by after services to pick up Noah for the day, and Brian, Abi, and I took a walk down to the cafeteria, stopping by the playroom on our way back for a change of scenery.

The next day approached us with a bang. It was Monday so Brian was back at work, and Noah was in school. I once again spent the night in Abi's room, each of us sleeping only four hours per the doctor's orders. The EEG was performed as scheduled, and we looked forward to being discharged the following morning. Since Abi and I were both exhausted from the previous night's lack of rest, we spent much of the afternoon napping in her room while waiting for Brian and Noah to arrive after work and school. Although I was on pins and needles wondering about the outcome of the EEG, I eagerly anticipated going home and moving forward, whatever that meant.

A New Medicine

The following morning, we were discharged and sent packing with a list of instructions and a new prescription. After being drug-free for nearly a full year, Abi would begin taking Trileptal. We began the dosing procedure that morning, and since it would take four weeks to reach what was called the "therapeutic level" of medicine in her bloodstream, we had to be on guard in case of further seizure activity.

Fortunately, this all came at the very end of the school year and Abi only had two weeks left before we had the entire summer to acclimate to life back on medication. Summer also served as the ideal time for Abigail to see various members of her medical team for follow-up appointments, minimizing her absences from school. We prepared for kindergarten by arming ourselves with information about her progress according to her medical professionals, as well as any changes in prognoses. This was helpful when we met with the IEP team at school to tweak her plan for the 2008–2009 school year.

Summer came and went, and before we knew it, the new school year was underway. With Abi being in a new class with a new teacher, there was a need once again to educate her as to what Abi's diagnoses and disabilities were. This meant a new IEP and materials to be handed to anyone who might interact with her while she was outside of my care. I developed the habit of composing notes for folks like the bus driver and PE teachers to inform them of Abi's delicate situation and the care involved, especially in case of a seizure in my absence. It was good practice, as the parent of a child with accommodations, to start the school year off by becoming acquainted with new teachers and establishing an open line of communication.

Since I was now subbing at school, I became more familiar with the staff and faculty, which only helped our situation. We seemed to once again be plugging along without any major upsets or changes in Abi's health, and I was again cautiously optimistic about her future.

Strides and Challenges

Abi made strides in the previous two years of preschool, having started out at the bottom of her class in terms of general skills and abilities, and progressing toward the middle by the beginning of her kindergarten year. Her first year of preschool, the teacher had characterized Abi as inconsistent and showing evidence of uneven processing skills and gaps in cognitive development. She missed a great deal of school due to doctor's appointments and hospitalizations, and I wondered how she would grow in development if that pattern were to continue. Placing this into perspective was a note on one of our correspondences with the school psychologist that Abi had missed fifteen of the past thirty-five days of school, which was both alarming and frightening to me. How could she ever be expected to get a quality education if this pattern continued?

Every one of the experts involved in Abi's case at school and at each of her medical specialists' offices warned us that her learning disabilities and delays would increase as the curriculum became more difficult. Knowing this, we anticipated that kindergarten would most likely prove to be her biggest challenge to date. Now that the medicine seemed to be controlling her seizure activity, and the side effects were minimal, I took comfort in the idea that at least medically, the worse part was behind us for now.

Abi's IEP was slightly revised for her kindergarten year, still focusing on speech therapy as the largest portion of the plan with 30 minutes a week of instruction. There would no longer be a need for physical therapy, and occupational therapy would only exist on a consultation basis. This was encouraging to me because the absence of necessary therapies and time out of the classroom setting meant progress in my mind. She would still have the sensory diet as part of her therapy, but the need would decrease as Abi became more comfortable in her new environment.

As time advanced, Abigail had setbacks both at school and at home, but her progress seemed to outweigh those setbacks, and I was fairly pleased with what we were seeing. She continued to struggle socially and seemed unable to adapt to new surroundings, but in a way that was not a distraction for herself or her classmates.

The meltdowns would come and go but seemed to take less time out of her daily routine. In the past she had difficulty resetting, as it would sometimes take her all day to come out of the funk that she would fall into over what seemed like insignificant occurrences to everyone but her. Now, I was pleased to see that she could reset her emotions within minutes of her breakdowns. I hoped that this would lead to new friendships with her classmates.

Although she was still behind her counterparts developmentally and academically, the gaps seemed to be smaller than they were during her two years of preschool. By the time that summer rolled around, I could look back on her kindergarten school year with gratitude and breathe a sigh of relief. Still, I knew that first grade would hold many challenges for Abi academically, and the curriculum would be significantly more difficult. Time would be our best indicator, but it also held many questions and much uncertainty.

To learn more about the medical terms and topics discussed in this chapter, visit this link:

www.SavingAbigailGrace.com

CHAPTER TWELVE

Seizures, Celebrations, and Saying Goodbye

AUGUST 2009 MARKED A MAJOR turning point for the Slaters. With Abi seeming to do fairly well and excited to begin her first-grade year, I felt it was safe for me to return to work full-time in order to ease our financial woes. After much debate, Brian and I decided it was time to close the business that we had been operating together for just under five years. He chose to go back to work as a financial advisor, and I happened to get a nice offer for an administrative assistant position downtown that would prove to be a fantastic experience for me, as well as provide a fair salary.

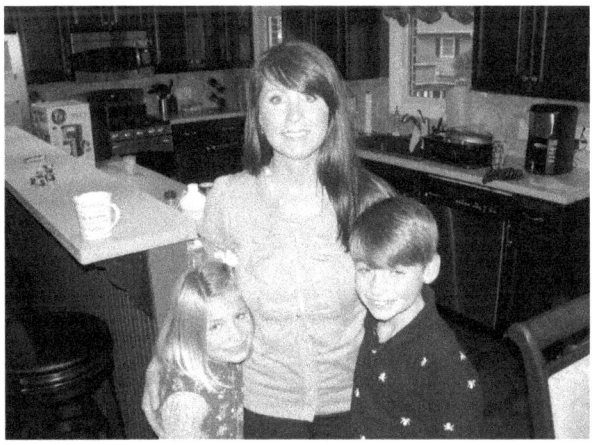

Our first day back to work and school

In fact, my first day at the new company was the kids' first day of school.

Staying Dry

As we moved into yet another year of school, Abi still struggled to stay dry during the times she slept. She and I were more frustrated than ever, wondering if she would ever see a night when she did not have to wear a pull-up to bed. I took her from one specialist to another, hoping we could cure her incontinence, but it was all in vain. To this day, if she misses a dose of her Desmopressin, she will be wet in the morning. But if that is the extent of her ailments after all she has been through, we both consider it a win!

We created a system where I would wake her up at night, right before I went to bed, and encourage her to use the bathroom. If she woke up with a dry pull-up the following morning, she placed a sticker on the calendar, indicating a major achievement for that day. This was an exciting process for her, and I noticed a change in the number of mornings that I had to strip her bed, bleach the plastic mattress cover, and launder her sheets—we were both encouraged. On mornings when she woke up wet, though she was disappointed, I made a conscious effort to celebrate the wins in hopes she wouldn't feel defeated.

Later, when Abi seemed to backslide in her progress using this system, we incorporated a bed-wetting alarm system into her nightly routine. I am sure that these alarms have improved greatly in the past fifteen years, but our experience was not great. It was an inconvenience to begin with, and the alarm scared the daylights out of our entire household when it alerted us to her bed-wetting.

Sometimes Abi would be in such a deep sleep that she wouldn't even wake up, while the rest of us scurried about the house like it was on fire. The alarm didn't last long, and given the price of the device, I was especially irritated when I had to store it along with other things we no longer used.

First Grade and Another IEP

As we did many times in the past, we sat down with the IEP team members at school to determine Abi's eligibility for services. Reevaluations were performed by several experts to gauge her progress and identify the areas where she still needed assistance. Evaluations and testing were conducted at the end of October, and we convened on November 10, 2009, with results and a revised IEP.

First grade was a bit more challenging for Abi than kindergarten, but she was fortunate to have the same teacher who had taught her during her two years of preschool. They had formed a special bond, and since this teacher was very familiar with Abi's medical history, learning challenges, and demeanor, I requested that she become Abi's first-grade teacher after hearing she had transitioned from preschool to first-grade.

With flaming red hair and the attitude to go with it, she was young, energetic, and had a strong desire to see all her students grow and achieve great things. She and I had always communicated well through preschool, and she treated Abi and me as part of the team instead of as intrusions into an otherwise perfect classroom, which I appreciated and really needed.

Another Seizure—The Worst One Yet

Abigail pushed through August and September like a champ in school and was doing well with her new and old friends. She had attended birthday parties and was still dancing and enjoying life as a typical six-year-old girl. On October 10, after seeing her neurologist for a routine appointment only three days prior, we ventured out of town for the weekend to spend time with friends, who lived about an hour and a half away from us. Our two families had a fun-filled weekend of partying with all five of our children, playing card games, eating lots of food, and laughing until we thought we would explode. On Sunday we packed our things into the vehicle, making our way back to Peoria.

Everyone was tired from the weekend's festivities, and we were looking forward to a casual Sunday at home with no plans except to lie about the house and do absolutely nothing. Over an hour into our drive, I happened to glance at the backseat to find that Abi was not behaving like herself. Both kids had been quiet, and I had been dozing in and out of a light sleep, assuming that they were doing the same.

Abi was sitting in the captain's chair of our SUV directly behind Brian's driver seat. When I looked at her, I noticed her left side was convulsing. Completely dazed with that "deer in headlights" look upon her tiny face, only her left eye was blinking, while the corner of her mouth was pulling to the left in unison. She was holding her left arm up in a 180-degree bend, and it was shaking at the same speed of the blinking eye and pulling lips. It all mimicked what I imagined a stroke would look like, but I knew in my heart that I was witnessing a seizure.

My first reaction, I am ashamed to say, was to freak out. This was the first time I had witnessed convulsions from her, and I was so scared that I started to shake with worry while yelling at Brian, who was now speeding down the highway toward the hospital. Up until this day, the seizures that I had witnessed looked more like daydreaming, and they were far less scary. "Brian! Oh my gosh, Abi's having a seizure! What should I do?" I cried, my voice escalating in volume with each word. "Just make sure you keep talking to her and calm down! I'm going to OSF," he answered in a very calm way, as was typical of him.

The convulsions were focused on her left side, while the right side was functioning properly. The craziest thing about this seizure was that Abi could have a conversation while it was occurring. Through tears, I asked her if she hurt anywhere, and she said her stomach hurt. Her voice was weak and puny, but I could understand her. She then asked me, "Mom, what is happening?" and I told her that she was having a seizure. "I'm scared," she said, and I told her that I was too, but that Daddy was driving us to the hospital. I timed her episode, which lasted approximately 13 minutes—quite lengthy for any epileptic event.

Meanwhile, Brian was hightailing it to the Children's Hospital Emergency Room like he was driving on a racetrack. I tried to remain calm, as he instructed me to do. All the while I just kept telling her, "It's okay, babe, it's all going to be fine. I'm here. Don't be scared. Daddy is getting us to your doctors," on repeat, and then, "Are you still feeling sick? Do you need to throw up?" And every few seconds, "You feeling okay? It's all fine babe, don't be scared."

Once at the hospital, Brian pulled the vehicle right up to the emergency door, flew out of his seat, opened Abi's door, and immediately scooped her into his arms. We all ran as if our lives depended upon it, scared and shaken by what we had observed. Noah ran after us, confused and worried about his little sister, but I was so devastated and caught up in my own emotions that the thought of comforting him never even occurred to me. I am lucky to have that sweet little man in my life; he never seemed to take it personally when our attention was focused on his baby sister.

Thrusting our way through the doors of the ER, we were immediately shown to a room where precautions were taken to create a safe environment for Abi. Her seizure did not cease until we were in the ER. After it ended, she was so tired that she could not keep her eyes open. The energy the seizure stole from her tiny body caused her to temporarily lose the ability to talk or answer any of our questions. Instead, she looked blankly at us as if she were not at all aware of her surroundings. The nurse asked her questions like, "What is your name?" and "Do you know where you are?" but she behaved as if she couldn't hear a word of it.

After having no verbal response, big, fat tears began to fall down her face, which told me that she could hear us and that she was scared. She was also likely frustrated by the fact that she was unable to respond with words. As I thought about what must have been circling through her complicated little brain, I could do nothing but weep alongside her. I felt hopeless once again, wondering and asking God, "Why? Why now? What did we do to deserve this?"

This had, by far, exceeded any scary circumstance I had faced since the accident that occurred nearly seven years earlier. I could hardly contain my emotions, and was ashamed of how I had come apart at the seams during such a time when I should have been more put together than anyone. After all, I was her mother, an adult, and she should have been able to find comfort in my presence, not fear. This would serve as a learning opportunity for us all, but for me, it also shook my self-confidence. I felt anything but strong in this situation, and while I was relieved that Brian was the rock upon which we all clung once again, I internally beat myself up with my thoughts.

A short time after her seizure ended in the ER, another episode took over Abi's body, this time as the medical staff watched and timed it. Thankfully, they were the experienced ones on the scene, and I was comforted by the idea that they knew what they were doing. This seizure lasted only a fraction of the previous seizure's length, but it seemed like an eternity as I could do nothing to help her. By the time it ended, Abi was completely exhausted and slept through being admitted into yet another room at Children's Hospital. *Here we go again*, I thought. "Please, God, I surrender." That was all the energy and courage I had to speak to Him.

Since Abi had been without seizure activity after starting medication during the last hospital visit, I was baffled by the day's events. She had had a fantastic weekend with friends, played to her heart's content, and no unusual activity had been witnessed by anyone around her. I wanted an explanation from those who knew best. I had so many questions and was completely on edge, thinking about the possibility that this could become an endless cycle for her and our family. When would this end? I thought we were on the other side of the yuck!

Unfortunately, with epilepsy, there are no clear-cut answers about the timing of an episode, so we had no way of knowing whether Abi would experience others. No one knows what triggers the onset of a seizure, and there is no way to anticipate one. This makes it tough to strike a balance between living one's best life and being too cautious to do anything but exist. I learned that there were dogs that could be trained to anticipate a seizure in patients lucky enough to adopt one. This was fascinating to me, and I vowed to research this option for Abi once we were back home from the hospital. At that point, though, I had no idea when that would be.

Once Abi was admitted to the main hospital and sleeping in her permanent bed, medical personnel of all sorts visited us. It was protocol for the neurologist and neurosurgeon to stop by each time we were admitted. To determine whether there was a shunt malfunction, or any changes since the last scans, they performed a CT scan of her head and a shuntogram. If there were changes, we might have answers as to why she had experienced what they call a "breakthrough seizure." It was called a breakthrough seizure simply because the episode occurred after being seizure-free for an extended period (at least 12 months) while taking the proper dosage of anti-seizure medication. This meant that the medicine was unable to control the seizures. Several factors could trigger these seizures, including sleep deprivation, severe stress, illness (especially infection and fever), and changes in blood sugar levels. In females, menstruation could even trigger breakthrough seizures because of the way our bodies react to the loss of blood and nourishment while we menstruate—something I would eventually have to watch for in Abi.

Each scan showed there had been no changes since the last and that everything appeared normal with the shunt. There had been no change in the position of her shunt, and it was functioning properly, indicated by the fact that there was no abnormality in the size of her ventricles and no overabundance of cerebrospinal fluid. Her head circumference was normal, indicating no swelling of the brain, and she was otherwise totally healthy with normal vital signs, so the question remained: Why did this happen?

There was no logical explanation for the breakthrough seizure, and after a brief two-day stay in our home away from home, we were discharged. Not wanting to risk another epileptic occurrence, Abi's neurologist decided to change her medication schedule, adding a new medicine called Depakene® to the Trileptal® she was already taking. This would, hopefully, minimize the chance of further seizures, but would undoubtedly cause side effects we would again have to manage.

Abi returned to school on October 13 but was sent home for behaving "oddly," as the school staff described. Her teacher, understandably nervous after hearing about our weekend, was afraid that Abi might be reacting to the effects of the new medicine. I, of course, picked her up and she stayed home for the rest of the week. I missed an entire week of work at my new job, giving Brian the ability to continue at his job, unaffected. While I was happy to be at home with Abi and provide her care, I had the most intense sense of déjà vu as my career again took a backseat to Brian's. It was terribly frustrating. With Saturday being Abi's seventh birthday, I was grateful that we were celebrating at home instead of in the hospital, even though the timing could not have been worse for her. Always find the silver lining!

A Chance to Educate

Seeing how nervous her teacher and some of the other staff were about Abi's seizure disorder—and being the mom who always wanted to educate others—I thought it would be invaluable to bring a specialist in to talk to the school staff.

Thankfully, when I raised the concern and suggested a solution (I was always taught to never complain without offering a solution) to the principal, she agreed to let me bring Abi's neurologist to a Teachers Institute, where all who attended would learn about epilepsy in a nutshell. Abi's neurologist arrived prepared with a slide show that focused on defining epilepsy, what it looked like, and what to do if a student ever suffered a seizure at school. It was remarkable how this short presentation seemed to put many of the teachers and staff at ease with seizures, and I felt more comfortable as a parent knowing they were better equipped. Abi's neurologist and I also distributed a "First Aid for Seizures" brochure published by the Epilepsy Foundation. This same illustration was part of Abi's insert that she always carried in her school binder.

Learning with Tutors

Slowly but surely, things became a bit more "normal" as Abi got back on track with school, allowing me to proceed with work as usual. We were beginning to see signs of what her medical experts had warned us might happen as her schoolwork became increasingly demanding. Preschool and kindergarten were challenging at times, but the curriculum was much more focused on socialization than on lessons of reading, writing, and arithmetic. First grade was proving to challenge Abi intellectually far more than she was prepared to endure.

As time progressed, we saw that her basic reasoning and problem-solving skills were underdeveloped at best. Reading comprehension was a subject in which she struggled greatly and would most likely always struggle. Her short-term memory failed her often, and as each school year passed, it became increasingly evident that it would be a lifelong labor for her. The part of the brain that was responsible for memory, as well as for problem-solving, had been severely damaged by the pooling of blood caused by the impact of the accident.

Although our brains have a way of compensating for such injuries, the tissue in this area of Abi's brain was, by all rights, killed off. Knowing this, there was little promise of these skills developing over time, and it is merely something she will contend with for a lifetime. Thankfully, she developed a love of reading books at an early age, and as she read on her own, I believe she exercised and strengthened her brain.

Math was more of an issue as the lessons became more difficult, and we continued to look for new programs that focused on math skills outside of Abi's classwork. This was a struggle, especially because she was already challenged during the day with various tasks at school, and then having to hurry home only to do more homework and attend more classes was utterly exhausting for her. We placed her in a program called Kumon that helped sharpen her math skills significantly, and took advantage of tutoring offered at our local Sylvan Learning Center.

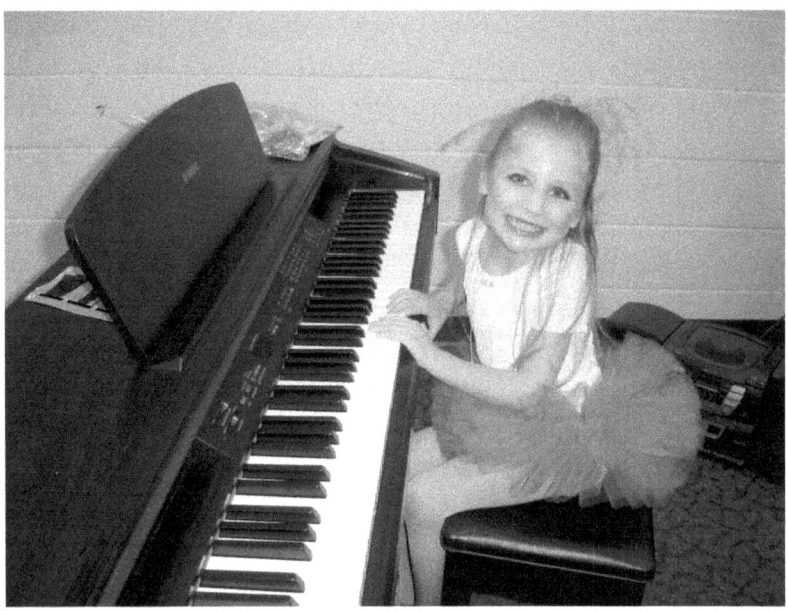

Two of Abi's favorite things: dance and playing the piano

Abi proceeded like the trooper she was, a complaint rarely leaving her lips. But because she was always tied up in her studies and homework, playtime with friends was becoming a rare occasion. Often, she would come home from school begging to play with a friend in the neighborhood only to be shot down because, by the time she finished her homework, there was no time. Twice a week she attended a math class after school and with dance and piano lessons, her life was much too structured at times. There seemed to be little time to enjoy the simplicity of childhood, and I constantly went back and forth between my feelings of guilt and sadness for her. It was difficult for me to let her be the little girl bottled up inside because I wanted her to be successful in everything she needed to accomplish.

Still, the extra time studying and attending classes outside of school seemed to pay off. By the time we sat down with her IEP team at school to prepare for second grade, it was determined that Abi would no longer qualify for the accommodations the IEP provided. The discussion instead revolved around the need for what they called a 504 plan. This plan included various recommendations for her in the classroom to help accommodate her learning disabilities. It is extremely important to know and fully understand the differences between an IEP and a 504 plan. There is a time and place for the 504, but I should never have allowed Abi to give up the accommodations of the IEP. You know what they say about hindsight and 20/20 vision.

Some of the recommendations to be implemented by Abi's teacher included checking frequently for understanding and making sure she stayed on task; providing preferential seating close to the teacher and quiet seating away from others, especially for test taking; reading tests aloud to an adult and retaking those she failed; highlighting important points while reading to assist in answering questions pertaining to the material; and displaying a visual schedule for her to refer to so she knew what to expect.

These accommodations were revised as needed from one year to the next. If the need ever arose for an IEP instead, that right would be given to her, provided she qualified according to the evaluations. When Abi made the transition from an IEP to a 504 I had mixed emotions, but knowing we could always request reevaluations in the future, my concerns were laid to rest, at least for the time being. I clung to that sheet of paper listing the accommodations and recommendations as if it were my last hope. It became my saving grace as Abi's advocate when new teachers entered the picture each year.

Although our experience with the school and its experts was generally a positive one, I became a very important advocate for my child. Without a plan in place and the relationships I built with everyone at the school, I question whether Abigail would have been as successful as she was.

I have seen many children not end up as fortunate as Abi was because their parents were not able to be as involved as I was. Some parents work multiple jobs to make ends meet and have no time to become heavily involved, as much as they may want to be. Others may not have the communication skills needed to contact the necessary adults, and simply do not understand the process. But, if you are able to make it work for your family, please get involved and stay involved in your child's life away from home. It could make all the difference for them.

RTI

Abi's grades didn't improve much, and as she graduated from second to third grade, I began to wonder if she would ever see an A or a B on her report card. Even with all the work both in and outside of school, her reports showed straight Cs nearly every grading period. Rarely would we see a B, and at times there were even Ds.

She had improved her math grade over time, but each time that occurred, it seemed to come at the expense to her reading grade. She became involved in a program at school that they called RTI, or Response to Intervention.

As time progressed, Abi was taken out of the classroom more and more for special reading and comprehension instruction. By the time she was in third grade, she had reached the need to participate in RTI for the maximum allowable time, which was one hour a day. This was great for accomplishing goals established for her reading and comprehension abilities, but not so great for the subjects that she was missing as a result.

Just as the law of physics suggests, for every positive action, there was an equal negative reaction. So while she was improving her reading skills, subjects like math and science became the proverbial thorn in her side.

Third grade brought about various feelings of defeat for me as Abigail's advocate and the one who devoted extra time to her cause outside of school. I felt I was constantly rubbing someone the wrong way, whether it was Abi's teacher or principal, and in my mind, the relationships that were strong in the past seemed to be crumbling. It was difficult to know how others perceived us, and maybe I had simply allowed my mind to play tricks on me, but I felt that some of those on Abi's team were growing tired of my questions, concerns, and overall presence. As much as I disliked that feeling at times, I had to remind myself that even if my feelings were valid, their annoyance with me was a necessary evil to get my daughter the care that she needed and deserved. Had I backed off and let nature take its course, I do not know if she would have achieved even a fraction of what she did. I stayed the course, focusing on growing a thicker skin, and not worrying whether others considered me a pest. I had to do what was right for Abigail.

Losing our Biggest Fan

Toward the end of Abi's third-grade and Noah's sixth-grade school year, my Superman dad became quite ill with bladder cancer. He had been "successfully" living with the affliction for about five years by then, but his health was steadily declining, unbeknownst to me. My family hadn't been completely forthcoming about his condition, and by the time I discovered how bad it had become, it was too late. Both he and Mom told me that they hesitated to "bother" me with the details because they knew how busy I was trying to keep my own family together, but it infuriated me when I heard those words. I'm not sure I ever forgave either of them for how they handled the whole thing.

My dad and I talked on the phone several times each week

while Mom was at work. She was still working full-time as a nurse after they relocated to southern Illinois years before, and Dad had retired before the move. He and I were having a typical conversation on the phone one day while he, as always, did laundry in the basement. I can still recall the conversation vividly, even after all these years. He was panting and out of breath from climbing the six stairs that led from the basement to their living room and started to make a choking sound that alarmed me. I immediately began to worry and asked, "Dad, what's going on? Are you okay?" He replied, "Layla, I'm not well. Hang on. . ." I heard the phone land on the ground as he threw up in the background. Tears fled my eyes, and my heart raced faster than ever. I felt dizzy and yelled into the receiver, "Dad, what is going on? You're scaring me!"

After his sickness subsided, he picked up the phone and simply said, "I'm dying, Layla." Oh God! This cannot be happening! No! No! No! "I'm coming down, Dad. Give me a few hours to get my things together, and I'll be there!" Of course, he tried to discourage me with his tiny whisper of a voice, but he knew it was no use. He knew me far too well to think he could keep me away, especially at a time like this. I frantically threw a few things into my overnight bag, called Brian at work to tell him what had just happened and that I would be gone for an unknown number of days, and off I went.

The drive from Peoria to Centralia was about three and a half hours, but it seemed to take days. I cranked up my music and lost myself in my thoughts, crying like a baby off and on until I pulled into my parents' driveway in their tiny town just off the two-lane highway. Dad had begun chemo, and I think somewhere in the back of my mind I knew that he would only slightly resemble the dad that would visit me in Omaha when Abi was in the NICU. But nothing in the world could have prepared me for what I was about to walk into. I opened the door to their living room from the front porch and grief smacked me in the face so hard that I thought I would fall to my knees.

My dad, once the most powerful man in my life—the one I always referred to as my Superman—now looked like a ghost of a human being. His oversized burgundy rocking recliner seemed to gobble him up. He looked incredibly thin and feeble, wearing his red St. Louis Cardinals stocking cap on his bald head and sitting cross-legged like a child. When had all this deterioration happened? I had been so busy with my own family that I had not given him enough time. Eyes sunken in and dark, he forced a toothless smile (his dentures no longer fit him) that almost immediately turned to a frown as he let the tears roll. Seeing him reduced to such a state knocked the wind out of me, but I found enough energy to drop down and hug him with all the force I could muster. *God, what have you done?* I thought to myself. *I thought you loved me. Why? Why him, and at this age?* My dad had just turned 61, and he would most certainly not live to see his 62nd birthday. Fury took over my body, and as ashamed as I was to feel this, I was powerless to control it. I was mad at God.

The house was an absolute wreck, which made me wonder what my mom and brother (who had lived with my parents until he had no choice but to leave years later) had been doing with their time. They had a Great Pyrenees dog named Gertie, and her hair was everywhere. The entire house looked like a cotton field because of it, and dirty dishes were piled sky-high. Being the person that I am, I began to frantically clean as if I was up against the clock—which, in a way, I was. I took care of Dad until Mom came home that evening to a newly cleaned house. We cooked dinner after catching up, but Dad, however hard he tried to eat, could not join us for our meal and remained in his recliner while Mom and I ate in silence.

I stayed for a few days and attended Dad's follow-up appointment in St. Louis with him and mom that week. We were anxious to find out if the chemo had worked and what the next steps would entail. We were not prepared for the emotional storm of that day. His doctor, after giving us the details of his findings (the chemo had not worked), propped his feet up on his desk and said, "Well, Gerry, it's time to call in hospice." Just like that! So nonchalantly, as if he were telling us the weather forecast. I was shocked, and honestly, wanted to punch the guy and watch him fall off that chair he was perched upon like a high horse. *You just handed my dad a death sentence, and you want to just kick back at your desk?* I thought.

My dad, sitting fraily in his wheelchair, simply said, "No shit?" And that was it. The beginning of a very short end to the life of the one man who never let me down. The one who loved my husband and kids as if they were his own. The man who, in his 61 years on this planet, never hurt anyone and would do anything for anybody. Unbelievable!

After the appointment, Mom and I packed Dad up into their vehicle, and she drove us back to Centralia. The mood inside their small SUV was somber, and the air felt so heavy it seemed like it could collapse my lungs at any moment. My breathing was labored, and I felt light-headed as I cried my eyes out, swearing to Dad that we would get another opinion. I had researched a facility in Chicago that I felt certain could save him, but he wouldn't hear of it. "I'm tired, Layla, and I couldn't make that drive; it would probably kill me," he said in response to my plea. "So you just want to give up? I don't get it. You're too young to die. Please just think about it, Dad." But there was no further response, and he drifted into a slumber for the rest of the car ride.

Metaphorically clutching my dad's death papers in my mind, I made plans to return home to gather my family for a trip that would be their final time seeing him alive. It was Easter when we returned, and we spent that time together, preparing ourselves for the inevitable. It was tricky trying to keep the mood somewhat light for my kids, who loved their grandpa. He was the only grandparent who truly engaged with them regularly. Historically, we would meet him at a halfway point during their school breaks, and he would take them to Centralia for a week at a time. In fact, that's how we ended up with the kids' first pet—a kitten that they found on the side of a road while visiting my parents. The black-and-white furball, who became known as Sox, made his way into our hearts and lived with us until he passed fourteen years later. They had a blast with their grandpa, who was like a kid himself, being active, especially outdoors with Gertie. He would take them fishing or to the park to play, just as he had done with my brothers and me when we were young. I don't know where he got his energy!

When the holiday was over, I said goodbye to Brian and the kids, and they said goodbye to Dad for the last time. I stayed behind to spend as much time with him as I possibly could, and to help Mom, who still needed to work. Because we had informed Dad's brothers and sisters of his condition, he took in many (sometimes unwanted) visitors over the next week, which exhausted him both physically and mentally. At one point, he asked me to take him up to his room, and when we got up there, we sat down on the edge of his bed. "Make them go away Layla. I can't handle it anymore," he said. I cried for a moment, then returned downstairs to where folks were gathered and politely asked them to leave. It was heartbreaking for me and for them, but I was there to make sure Dad was comfortable and to grant him any last wishes.

We watched that sweet man become a pile of bones until he took his final breath on May 1, 2011, while my mom, youngest brother, and I willed him to join his loved ones in Heaven. By that time, he couldn't speak because his lungs had filled with fluid, and as though scripted from the most heart-wrenching movie, he exited this world with a single tear streaming down his face. My world came to a screeching halt, and nothing has been the same since. Mom never recovered. He was the love of her life, the only man she ever loved, and she was lost without him by her side.

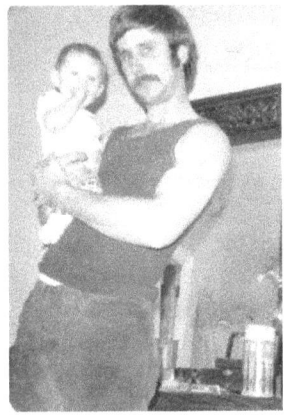

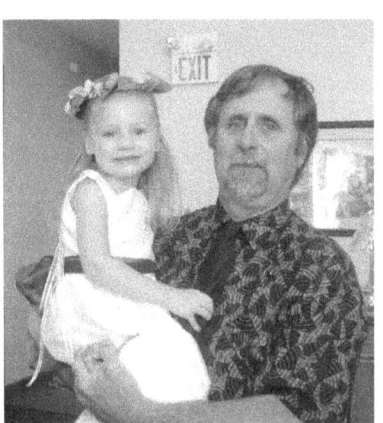

Young me with my dad (left) and young Abi in the same pose, about 30 years later (right)

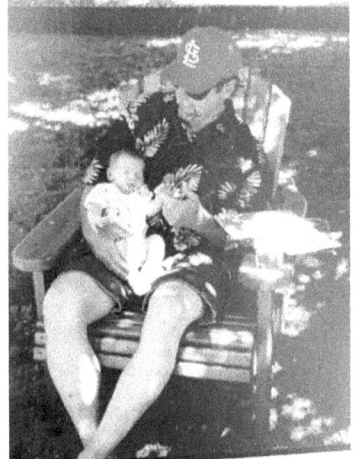

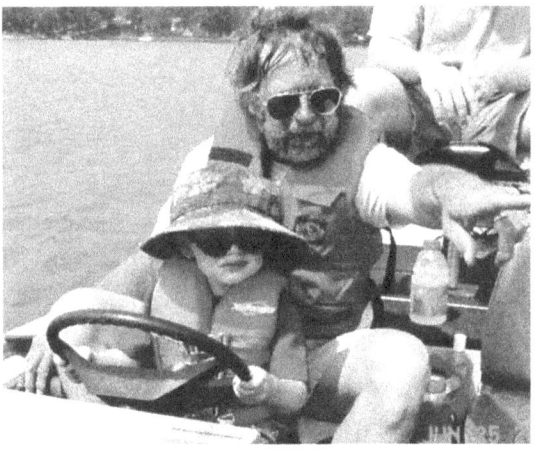

Dad with baby Noah

Dad in his element, teaching Noah about boating and fishing

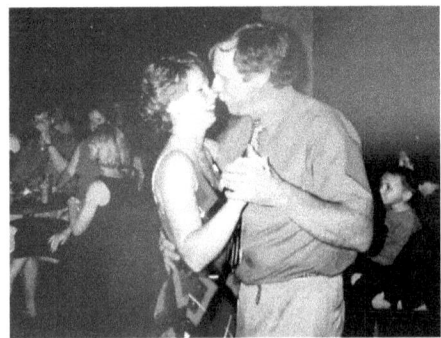

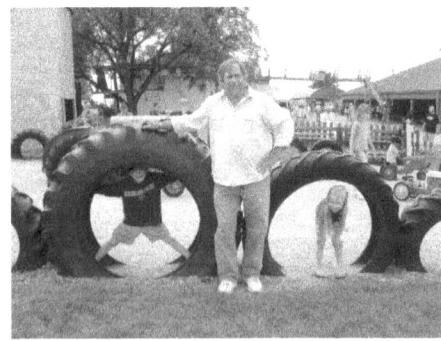

Dad and me at my wedding reception

Dad was the best Grandpa!

Once Dad's memorial was over, and we were all back in Peoria, trying to get back to our routines, I felt a dark cloud following me everywhere I went for months. I couldn't shake it no matter how much I prayed for it to go away. Some days, all I could do was cry; other days, I would feel totally fine. The depression was so bad that my body hurt all the time, the kind of hurt that happens the day after your hardest, most labor-intensive workout. My mom was much worse for wear, and I worried she might take her own life. Being far away from her during her darkest days made my heart ache, but I was always just a phone call away. Brian, Abi, and Noah needed me too, and my life was in Peoria, so I did the best I could to put one foot in front of the other each morning when I crawled out of bed. Eventually, things became easier.

Back to Reality

Brian did an amazing job keeping up with everything on the home front in my absence, but jumping back into my role was a necessary distraction from my own grief. After the fog from my dad's passing had cleared a bit, we all resumed our regular routines the best we could with summer break approaching. Seeing what being involved in a plethora of extracurricular activities was doing to Abi's mental state, I took time before the new school year to reevaluate. As her hatred for math grew, I decided that the extra math class at Kumon would have to subside for now. During the first part of third grade, she was not only attending that class and doing the homework required seven days a week, but she was also seeing a math tutor twice a week after school. It was just too much for her to bear, and it was unfair for her to be overwhelmed all the time by work. I had to make a change for the sake of her sanity.

Abi was no longer involved in dance but was still taking piano lessons. After discussing it with her, we concluded that her weekly half-hour lesson was a much-needed break in her week, so we kept that on the itinerary. I gave her permission to just do the best she could with practicing piano during the week, and if she did not feel up to it every day, it was no big deal. This proved to be a good decision because it served as a creative outlet for her, while strengthening her left hand and fingers and working her brain in parallel with her academic studies. Piano was a win-win for Abigail.

By January 2012, she was involved in RTI for an hour each day during school, saw her math tutor twice weekly for hour-long sessions after school, and attended piano lessons once a week for half an hour, practicing at her leisure. In addition, I worked with her math and reading teachers to have copies of worksheets for her to complete at home in place of the math homework that we had eliminated with the after-school math class.

Although I initially made this part of her home study a daily requirement, I adjusted it weekly according to her homework load, being careful not to overwhelm her.

All seemed to work to her benefit, and there was some improvement in her overall attitude toward life in general, her schoolwork more specifically. She was able to socialize a bit more than she had in the past, achieving more of a balance between work and play time. Her math grade fluctuated between a B and a C, while her reading grade bounced around from a C to a D. I learned to live with it as long as I felt we were doing everything we could do, and as long as she was giving it her best effort.

Now that she was in fifth grade, I decided it would be best to have her reevaluated for the purpose of replacing her 504 plan with a fresh IEP that could grow with her from one grade to the next. After requesting a conference and consenting to the reevaluation in November 2013, Abigail underwent evaluations with the district's psychologist, social worker, and the school's special education team. By December of that same year, she had a new IEP. That IEP served as legal documentation of her rights to certain accommodations throughout her entire classroom experience in grade school, middle school, and high school. To this day, Abi still uses many of these accommodations and has become a strong self-advocate.

Middle School

In middle school, Abigail chose to follow in her athletic brother's footsteps and participate in running cross country. Remember the girl who had a tough time using her left side as a little tyke? Well, that girl ran miles alongside her peers on the team and excelled at cross country as well as track. It was fun to watch her and Noah compete in the same events, sometimes at the same time, and school athletics kept us quite busy from 2013 through Abi's high school graduation in 2021.

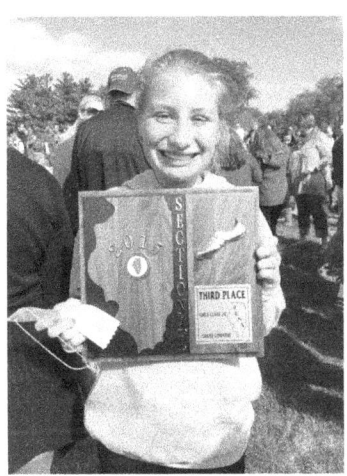
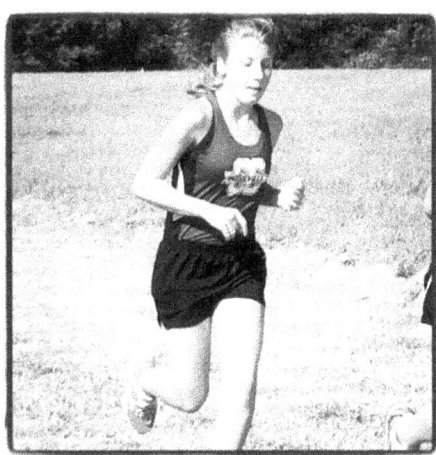

Being seizure-free since her hospitalization in 2009 and finally finding the right medication and its therapeutic dose—as well as having a solid IEP in place—led to a somewhat uneventful few years. Her EEG and MRI from July and August of 2011 proved to be what her specialists called "unremarkable," a term that we loved to hear regarding her medical history! While there was still evidence of abnormalities in her brain waves, the EEG showed "no electrographic or electrocortical seizures," and her MRI showed "no evidence of hydrocephalus or acute intracranial abnormalities". Praise God!

While Noah was three grades ahead of Abi in school, and because their school building was a K–8 setting, there was one year that both kiddos were in track and cross country together. Those days were incredibly fun and busy, and we never missed a meet. Noah was an exact replica of his dad and was naturally talented in sports, while Abi wasn't participating so much for the competition as she was to simply stay active with her big brother. She looked up to him in every way, and seeing them run alongside each other brought me a level of joy I couldn't begin to describe.

Noah was also involved in concert band and jazz band from fifth grade through high school as a drummer, which tested our patience more times than not. While he was just beginning to learn his instrument, we thought we would lose our minds some nights as he banged away with seemingly no purpose. But we were happy to support him and watched him grow into quite an incredible musician. Once he reached high school, he would also join the marching band and drumline, and we very much enjoyed attending his performances.

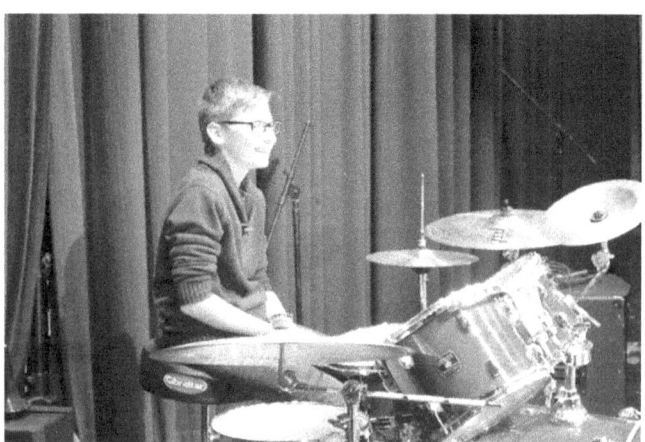

Noah on his drum kit at a Jazz concert

Urology

Because Abi was still struggling to stay dry during the night if she missed a dose of Desmopressin, her pediatrician referred us to a pediatric urologist with hopes to rid her of the "nocturnal and diurnal enuresis." They found that her organs were perfectly developed and functioned properly, so she began physical therapy to strengthen the pelvic floor muscles and to learn how to drain her bladder when she used the bathroom. She was also put on a MiraLAX regimen, and we were instructed to analyze her stools. The urologist wrote a note for the teachers to keep in their classrooms, excusing her to use the bathroom at regularly scheduled times (10:00 a.m., noon, and 2:00 p.m.), allowing her the chance to empty her bladder throughout the school day. Otherwise, my timid wallflower would wait until the last minute to ask to use the restroom, not wanting to interfere with classroom instruction and call attention to herself. Sometimes this led to accidents, requiring me to bring her fresh clothes. We quickly learned that being proactive and leaving fresh clothes and undergarments in her school locker would prove valuable and save her from an awful lot of embarrassment.

After going back and forth with the urology department and the physical therapist, trying exercises and dietary/supplement changes, we finally learned that the enuresis had nothing to do with her bladder or her waste excretion habits. Instead, the neurologist told us that there was a disconnect happening inside her brain that would likely prove to be a permanent struggle for her without medication. Even as an adult, she still takes Desmopressin every night before bed to prevent bed-wetting. While this is an inconvenience for her, we are reminded that her situation could be much worse.

In July 2013, after careful consideration and discussion with Brian and me, Abigail's neurologist decided that we would wean her from Trileptal since it had been four years since her last seizure. We were cautiously optimistic and excited for Abi since this meant the only medicine, she would continue to take was Desmopressin. I am beyond grateful to be able to report that, after being seizure-free for nearly 15 years and free of seizure meds for nearly 10 years, Abigail is thriving as a college student and still only takes Desmopressin for nocturnal enuresis. What a fantastic accomplishment!

Living the School Activities Life

Abi was baptized at a local non-denominational church on January 29, 2012, where we were attending church services as a family. The kids loved their children's church activities, met many new friends, and grew with them in Christ. I became heavily involved, once again, in volunteering at the church, and Brian and I occasionally attended small group Bible study sessions.

Noah had been baptized years earlier at the Baptist church we attended for years, and Brian and I were baptized in Brian's childhood church many years apart. Being a Christian, my mind and soul were set at ease once we had all accepted Christ and were baptized.

We were grounded in our faith and focused on school activities as Noah became more involved in band and choir, as well as track and cross country. He always excelled with ease at his schoolwork and athletics, made friends easily, and breezed through life effortlessly, which was a blessing for us all. I think God knew that I could only handle one kiddo that needed extra attention, so he put Noah on cruise control through Abi's toughest years. We rarely had to help him with his homework, thankfully, because he always seemed to take tough courses.

While Abi was plugging away in middle school, Noah was doing the same in high school, keeping us busy with school friends and volunteering at concession stands and wherever else the sports and band boosters needed us. I volunteered as a band mom, taking on various roles as we traveled each weekend to other small towns where football and marching band were a way of Friday-night life. Since Noah was in the marching band during the cross-country season, there were weekends when we wouldn't see our friends at all unless they were also band or cross-country parents.

With Abi in middle school and Noah in high school, no longer on the same teams, we accepted the "divide and conquer" lifestyle for several years. Like many parents of involved youngsters, our days consisted of working our 8-to-5 jobs, and picking up the kids from practices, or attending meets and performances. Our old friends took a backseat to the friends of convenience that we hung around for the sake of the kids. This was the season of the kiddos and, knowing that one day we would get to discover our own season, we were more than happy to assume the roles given to us.

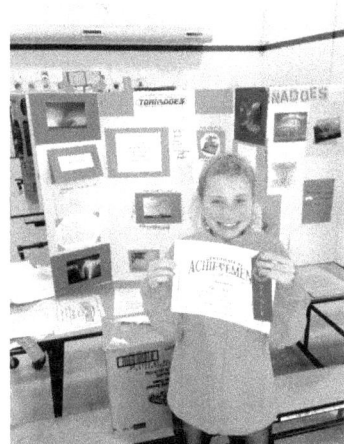
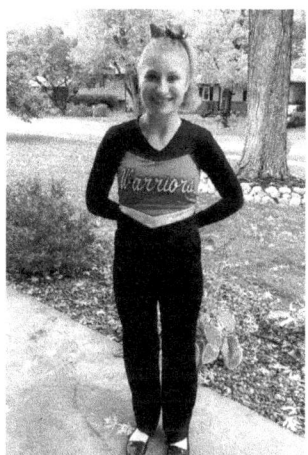

The kids volunteering at Peoria Family House

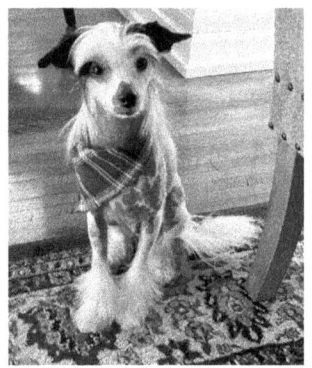
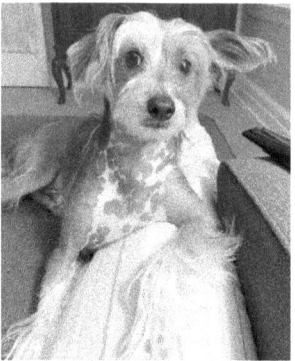
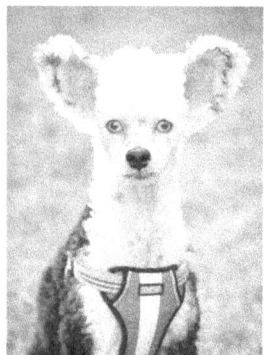

Bentley   *Rambo (BoBo)*   *Loki*

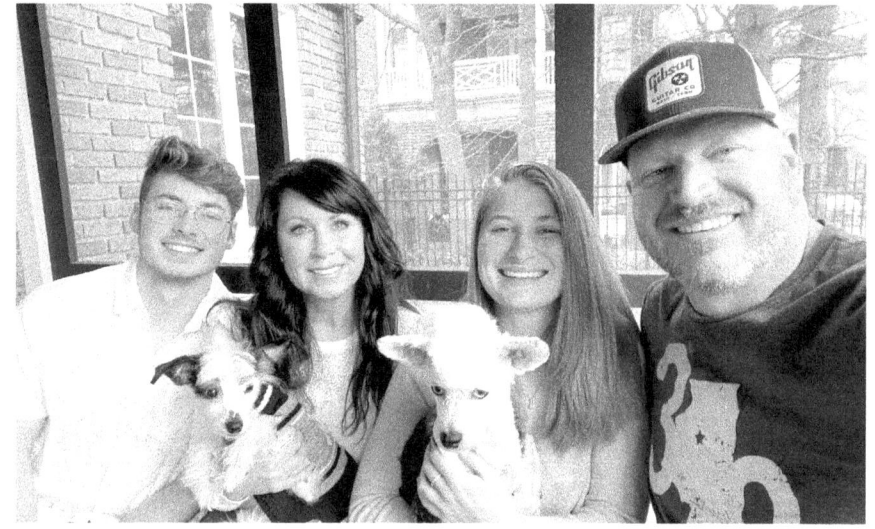

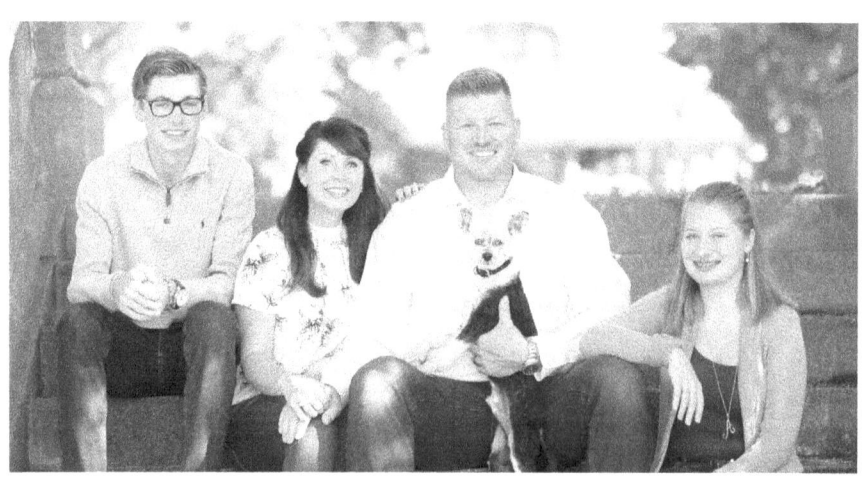

Our Family Grows in a Canine Direction

We bought our first dog while the kids were teenagers, and he came to us via air from the breeder in March 2016. I had always loved the Chinese Crested breed and we found a black-and-white one of the Powder Puff variety in Missouri with whom I instantly fell in love. Loki was full of energy—to the extent that the breeder, as she sent regular videos of him and his siblings, referred to him as a "crackhead." The love he brought into our home was like nothing we had ever experienced with an animal before. Of course we had our rescue kitty, Sox (who Mom always said was sent to us from Heaven, even though she knew I was allergic), but I never felt as close to him, and he really ended up being more Noah's cat than the family's.

Since I have a profound love for Chinese Cresteds, I bullied Brian into allowing me to adopt a little five-year-old brown-and-white hairy hairless dude named Rambo in 2018. He was a scrappy guy, all fourteen pounds of him, and had zero patience for any human. The poor little man had been neglected in his previous years and his teeth and nails had begun to rot away (we found out later that he had some type of autoimmune disease). His favorite pastime was biting people on their backside, with a preference for large ones. Our house guests never seemed to like him for some reason, but as mean as he could be, he was my little shadow. I couldn't go anywhere without him walking along beside me, and I was so in love with him and his nutty personality that when we had no other choice but to put him down two years after we adopted him, I fell apart.

Losing a pet is one of the toughest things to endure. We had a connection like no other, and I was lost without him. Not to take away from my bond with Loki, who I love dearly, but there was something about Bo that was just different. Brian and Noah buried him in our backyard, beneath the hammock where Abi still loves to read her books in the summertime.

Sox passed away one year after Bo did, in 2021, leaving both kids, especially Noah, incredibly sad. He was Noah's buddy for fourteen years, and Noah really couldn't remember a time before Sox quite literally fell into our family. We called him home from school on that rainy day so he could bury him right beside Bo in our backyard.

When Bo passed away, I became fixated on the idea of adding another hairy hairless Crested to our family so that Loki could have another furry friend. When I found a like-minded Crested owner on Instagram whose dog had new pups, I reached out to her. Born in September 2021, we were blessed with Bentley and made arrangements to meet his owner in Chicago to pick him up just before New Year's Eve of the same year. Abi says that I had to get another creature to care for since both of my human children deserted me, which is probably true. Once a mom, always a mom, right?

Whatever the reason, Bentley completed our new nest, and we now take our two canine boys with us everywhere we travel.

Saying Goodbye to Mom

Mom had all but given up on living the day that my dad left us seven years earlier. She tried to find joy from time to time, but even on her best day while Dad was alive and well, she struggled with depression and anxiety. I'm not sure exactly when she became depressed, but it was sometime during my high school years. She had always wanted to be nothing more than a wife and a mom, and she was great at both roles while we were young. My childhood is full of beautiful memories, like those of her singing in the most angelic voice while she was learning to play guitar. My parents were active with us three kids when we were growing up, but once I was in high school and learning to spread my wings, things began to go south for Mom.

My middle brother and I are only 15 months apart in age and were in high school together for three years. The pain she felt when we no longer depended on her for our every need was more than she could bear. I remember on several occasions finding her in bed in the middle of the afternoon when

I returned home from school, many times with a tear-soaked pillow beneath her weeping head. With Dad golfing almost every day back then and we kids living our own lives, she felt betrayed by us all. Over the years she would experience very high highs and even lower lows, to the point that she was always on some anti-depressant. It never seemed to work, though.

For some reason, she never allowed herself to become immersed in the lives of her kids or grandkids the way Dad did. When he died, all the birthday cards inscribed with his crazy poems stopped coming. She called sometimes, but cried through most conversations, and whenever I called her, it always seemed to be a bad time. I tried to help her in any way I could, but she was far enough away geographically that I couldn't do for her what I wished I could. She and I had such a complicated relationship once I grew into an adult, that it took a lot out of me to try to please her, especially when I knew there was no way to do it with any consistency.

When Brian earned a trip with his employer to London, he asked me if I wanted to take Mom and make it what he visualized as a life-changing family vacation. Maybe this experience would be the one that would breathe new life into Mom and shed some much-needed sunshine on her dark world. Since his employer was paying for much of his portion of the trip and part of my attendance, we felt we could afford to take Mom and the kids. While we planned the details of the vacation, we found that adding a few days in Paris to the itinerary would also be "affordable"—a small fortune we were willing to part with—so we added three days and two nights to the front end of the trip.

We called Mom and pitched our plan and itinerary to her, practically begging her to join us, and she reluctantly agreed. It was settled! The five of us would spend Christmas and New Year's Eve in the UK!

On Christmas Day 2014, we all boarded a plane in Chicago and headed east, "across the pond," to have the most unforgettable vacation ever. After a very long day of traveling, we landed in

Paris and hit the ground running, not wanting to waste a single second of exploring the City of Love.

Because it was Christmas, the city was quiet, but we managed to find a café that was open near our hotel and drank our first Parisian cappuccinos. I felt like I was drinking from a coffee fountain in Heaven—it was the most delicious coffee I had ever tasted! The folks who took care of us there spoke enough English, and we spoke enough very broken French, that it was a perfect way to begin our trip. Mom was exacerbated by the flights but still managed to at least behave as though she was having a nice moment.

The following night, after exploring the city like children at the North Pole, we all embarked on a dinner cruise that I had booked months before. The landing from where we boarded the all-glass vessel was at the foot of the Eiffel Tower, and the entire area on each side of the River Seine was oozing with Christmas spirit. Lights hung from every tree, and we witnessed, as a family, for the first time, the magic of the twinkling Eiffel lights of which I had only heard before that night. It was such a brilliant spectacle—so awe-inspiring that even my stoic mother oohed and aahed, her eyes dancing with wonder.

Once aboard the ship, Brian, Mom, the kids, and I enjoyed the most incredible meal that any of us had ever tasted! Each course was accompanied by a perfect wine pairing, presented with such confidence and grace by our wonderful servers. (The kids had their choice of beautifully presented, kid-friendly beverages with fruit garnishes.) Before this trip, I had imagined that this Parisian experience would be filled with dream-worthy enchantment, but it was more than I ever could have anticipated. To this day, despite traveling to many parts of the world, it is unmatched.

Once we had consumed all the calories that our bellies could possibly allow, we ended the dining experience with more cappuccinos, created in the signature Parisian way, that were both picturesque and delicious. Mom, who almost never partook in beverages of an alcoholic nature, enjoyed enough wine to invoke incredible carefree laughter. As we trekked back to our hotel on foot, she locked arms with me in a way that made me believe the trip could indeed be a turning point for her and for our relationship.

We spent the rest of our time in Paris walking in wonder through every part of the city, taking in all the beauty that it had to offer during the holiday season, and then we made our way to London via the Eurostar train. While at the Paris Gare du Nord train station, I watched my mother revert to the woman we knew in the US—somber, anxious, and withering like a fern in direct sunlight. What the locals called gypsies canvassed the station and its surroundings, approaching us all for money and tugging on our clothes when we tried our best to ignore them. It was more than my mom could handle and before we knew it, she was so upset that she wouldn't even attempt to complete her own immigration forms. Brian was forced to do it for her while I completed mine and the kids' forms.

London was an amazing experience, as none of us had been there before. Since we were technically there for Brian's work trip, we did have a small number of gatherings with other financial advisors that we were required to attend. The company set up unique tours and experiences for everyone, which took the busy work off our plates and allowed us to just take it all in. Being huge Harry Potter fans, we were blessed with a full day at the Harry Potter Universal Studios set, where much of the movies were filmed, and Mom enjoyed that. We spent New Year's Eve at Madame Tussaud's Wax Museum and once again witnessed a light-hearted, fun-loving version of Denice Paulus, champagne in hand. But most of the week, when I expected to enjoy sightseeing, Christmas lights and decorations, and once-in-a-lifetime experiences with my whole family, Mom became increasingly distanced and quiet.

By the time we boarded the homeward-bound plane after our 10-day stay abroad, Mom was barely speaking to any of us.

Brian's and my plan to restore joy into her life had shattered. Once we were back in Illinois, after she spent the night at our place before heading back to her home, it was painfully clear to me that we would never again know the Denice that existed when I was a child. She would spend the rest of her days wishing for the Lord to "take her home" where she would reunite with the love of her life. That hurt us all to our core, and I especially felt like the sword that had pierced my heart years before had finally bled it out.

Mom was diagnosed with breast cancer in 2015, and once she seemed to beat that, she was diagnosed with lung cancer. She had always been a smoker, so I suppose it was inevitable that the cigarettes would be responsible for ending her life prematurely.

She endured chemotherapy and radiation for breast cancer and then underwent a bilateral mastectomy with reconstruction of each breast. After such an intrusive surgery, she became extremely ill. Her doctors discovered an infection where the implants were placed, and eventually, they removed them, replacing them later with a second set. This was an incredibly tough time for her and for my brothers and me. After all her illnesses and treatments, she was still hopelessly addicted to cigarettes. This addiction, paired with her refusal to nourish her body with healthy foods, made her healing process long and treacherous. She also took an early retirement from her job as a nurse, and I believe that was a major blow to her sense of self-worth.

Mom eventually overcame breast cancer, but in 2018 was diagnosed with lung cancer. By that time, she had all but given up fighting against the inevitable, but she endured yet more chemotherapy and radiation, all the while continuing to smoke. Because she had been a nurse for so many years, I found it difficult to understand how she could continue to make unhealthy food and habit choices. I was beyond frustrated with her. I encouraged her to eat healthy, cancer-fighting foods and made superfood smoothies when I visited, but she hated them, complaining that they "tasted like dirt." While I was trying my best to nourish her body, friends and past coworkers were dropping by with all the sugar the house could store, with the best intentions, of course.

Mom's oncologist finally decided that the time had come to transition her to hospice care, which would be provided in her home. My brothers and I clung to the hope that a miracle could still happen, but it was another sharp punch in the gut for us all. Once again, seven years after doing this with Dad, we welcomed hospice workers, a hospital bed, and all the fixings that come along with it, into Mom's living room.

During the short time that she was in hospice care at her home in southern Illinois, I took on a role much like the one I assumed when Dad was dying. I spent a great deal of time away from my family, my work, and my town while I assumed the role of caregiver to my last surviving parent. I would never wish that kind of pain on anyone—watching a parent slip away while you are helpless.

She didn't go in the same manner that Dad went. While he mostly passed peacefully over the few weeks that he was in hospice care, my mom fought it with every bit of strength she could find. Not even the heaviest doses of morphine and fentanyl would keep her comfortable. It was torture to watch her attempt to climb out of bed using her bony arms and legs to flail herself over the metal railing. My brother and I had to barricade her with chairs and sleep at her bedside to make sure she didn't hurt herself.

Mom was convinced during that time that she was going to Hell, not Heaven, and she would scream and cry and ask for forgiveness at all hours of the night. My heart felt like there were shards of glass scraping against its insides, and I spent many sleepless nights doing all that I could to soothe her. My brothers and I called upon several men of God, all from different faiths, to come over and talk to her about why she believed she was unworthy of Heaven. She seemed to feel at ease as they were there, but as soon as they left, she would torture herself again.

We also called her cousins, Robbie and Juie, who were raised with the same spiritual beliefs as she was, in hopes that they could talk her through this troubling thought process, but it really never subsided. In my mind, Mom was as near to perfect as a human could get, so I was puzzled by her behavior. While my brothers and I were children, she was an amazing mother whose only focus was on us and my dad. Her faith in God was always strong, even if she did not attend church, and she prayed often. She stood by her values and beliefs and lived according to the teachings of the Bible, giving herself only to my dad and keeping her vows— "till death do us part." Mom was honest, stayed away from gossip, drank alcohol only on rare celebratory occasions, and never even got a speeding or a parking ticket. How could she possibly be so tormented while God was preparing her space in His kingdom?

My youngest brother, who still lived with her, lacked patience and often tried to force her meds down her throat while yelling at her. As a result, he and I found ourselves at each other's throats quite often. Meanwhile, Abi's birthday party, that I had planned for her and her new classmates, was approaching. I decided on a Friday, after a terribly rough night, to leave Mom's place and return on Sunday. My plan was to throw Abi the best party I could throw on that Saturday so that she wouldn't feel overlooked, after which I would drive back to relieve my brothers. I prayed all the way home that she would hang on until I returned.

On the day of Abi's party, while I was knee-deep in birthday decorations and planning the best weenie roast I could possibly pull off under the circumstances, my brother called me with news I somehow knew I would get from afar. I can't explain it, but I had a gut feeling when I left Mom's house that she would finally let go once I was back in Peoria. She almost seemed to be waiting for me to leave so that I wouldn't be there to witness her departure from this world, and that thought plagued me.

Mom passed on the day of Abi's party, October 26, 2018, at just 64 years old.

Maybe it was largely the suffering imposed by her broken heart that caused her to give up the ghost, just weeks before Noah was sworn in at Jefferson Barracks as an Airman of the United States Air Force. She and Dad would both have been deeply proud of him for committing his life to serving, especially since my dad and my middle brother served in the army.

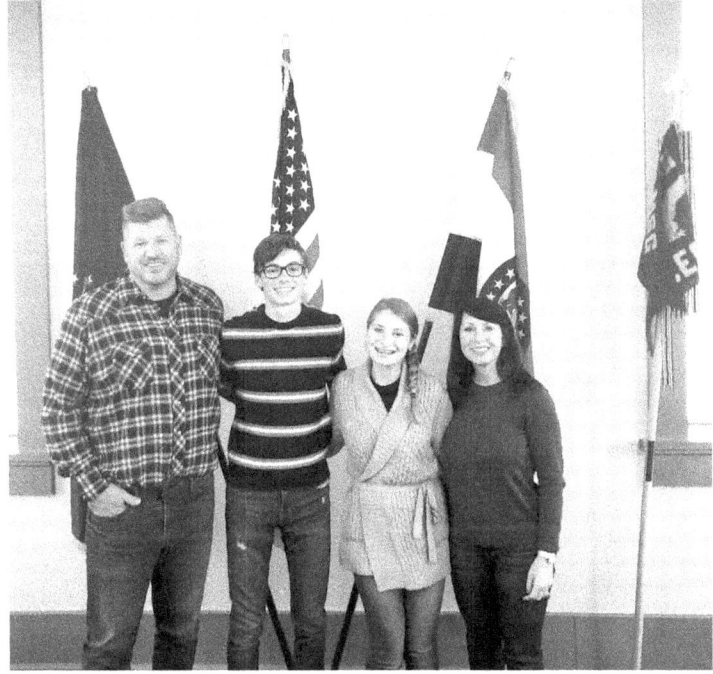

Noah's swearing-in at Jefferson Barracks

With both my parents, the only grandparents who were ever truly involved with my kids, now in Heaven, my extended family was in pieces. But my focus has been—and always will be—on my own children and my husband, just as the Bible tells us it should be.

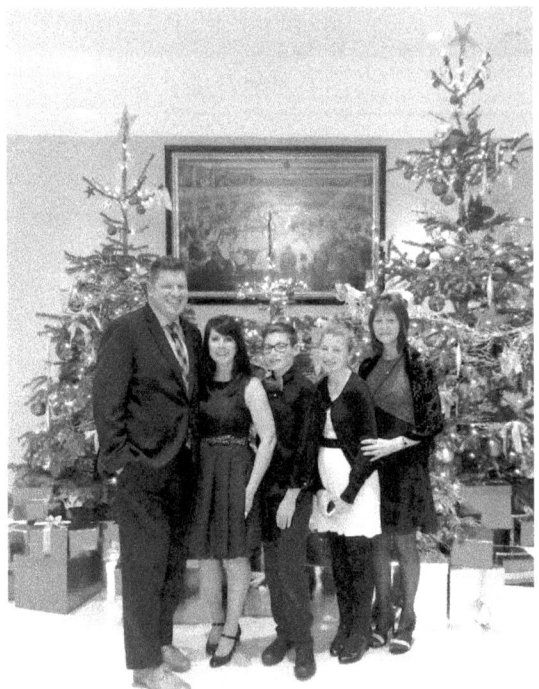
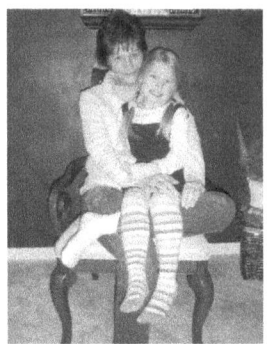
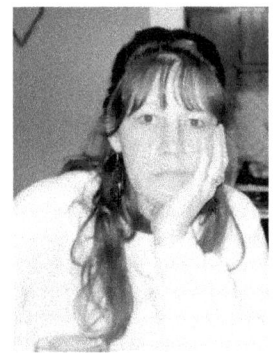

To learn more about the medical terms and
topics discussed in this chapter, visit this link:

www.SavingAbigailGrace.com

CHAPTER THIRTEEN

Growing Forward and Healing Together

High School and Beyond

Abi cruised through middle school and became heavily involved in extracurricular activities like choir, cross country, and track. As I think back to the difficulties she had when she was learning to ride her bike and swim because of her left-sided cerebral palsy, it is that much more incredible to know that she could excel at sports. Once she was in high school, she even decided to join the swim team and proved to be quite good at the sport. She was the poster child for what hard work, determination, and lots of prayers can do for a person.

Although Abigail was experiencing improvements in her medical journey, school was still proving to be quite difficult for her, and making solid friendships was simply not happening. One thing her specialists warned us about was that she would likely ex-

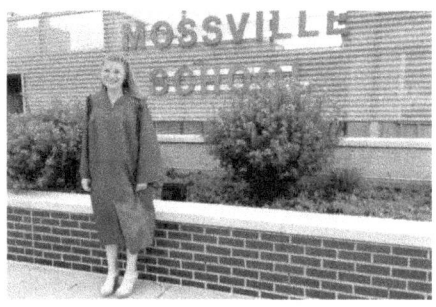

Abi's 8th grade graduation

perience manipulation and bullying since she was less capable than the average person of making wise decisions and standing up for herself. Children who are "different" from others can become prey to those who sense weakness, and her sweet spirit was taken advantage of more than occasionally. She struggled sometimes with finding her own self-worth and feelings of inadequacy, especially as a teenager.

She was also a transfer student in high school when we moved back to Peoria the summer that she went into her sophomore year. She transferred from a school district where everyone knew her and her family, to a private Catholic school where nobody knew us at all. This move was not one that we had planned for a long time, and we did not take it lightly, as it was an opportunity to buy a beautiful historic home that seemed meant to be. We considered all the pros and cons before we made our decision, and since Noah had already graduated from high school and was attending a local community college, we felt it was as good a time as any. But there were major struggles with Abi's new school for which we could not have adequately prepared.

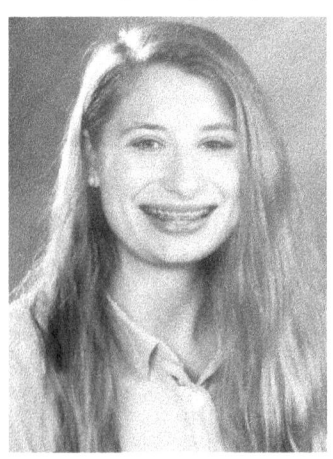

Although we were not Catholic, we chose to place Abi in a Catholic high school after touring it and a Christian high school. The Peoria public high school would not have been the best choice for her, so we scraped the money together to pay for private tuition, where we knew she would have a chance to learn without the distractions that came with the public school that she otherwise would have been forced to attend. One problem with this was that private schools had different standards, at least in the state of Illinois, for IEP equivalents (called ISP in the private setting) than public schools.

While we still would meet with the public district's special education team, the staff at the private school were not as equipped to accommodate children with learning disabilities.

Although we were fortunate enough to have an overall wonderful experience with our previous public school district in terms of their staff and administration accommodating Abi, the private school provided quite a different experience. There are obvious differences between a public school's IEP and a private school's ISP, and these differences are based primarily on funding.

While public schools typically have a strong budget for special education services because they are state funded, many private schools do not. They may be able to use some of the school district's resources at times, but it is not a guarantee and especially depends upon the state and local regulations.

Where an IEP is a legal document that can continue seamlessly from one school year to the next, an ISP's continuity is not guaranteed. If the funds are not available during a particular school year, the student can lose services such as PT, OT, speech therapy, and other costly services. This can be devastating for students who depend upon these services and can force families to seek such services privately outside of school hours, which can be quite costly and sometimes downright unaffordable.

And finally, at least in our particular experience—because it seemed the majority of the students at Abi's private high school were exemplary students, at least academically— teachers either did not have the patience for those who struggled academically or did not have the necessary tools. There were several instances where this became evident, and since I taught Abi to advocate for herself, it was tough for me to let her do that while I sat in the background. The private high school was focused on a college-preparation curriculum, so the material was significantly more challenging than that of the high school from which she transferred.

Abigail did a fantastic job advocating for her accommodations, but not every teacher was on board. Some of them would deny her accommodations, such as being able to take her quizzes and exams in an alternate location or being granted extra time to finish assignments, projects, quizzes, and exams, because they felt it was "cheating." And because she was a sophomore in high school, I tried desperately to let her fight her own battles. Nonetheless, there were times when I got involved because I felt she was being taken advantage of or not given the benefit of the doubt because of her medical history.

Abi's Friendships

Abi also had a tough time making friends at this school, because all the kids had grown up together in the same local Catholic elementary or middle schools. The only kids that seemed to be open to new friendships were those who didn't have friends to begin with, for reasons that became obvious to us as we learned more about them.

When Abi was a new student at the high school, knowing nothing of the other students other than what she saw for herself, she ended up surrounding herself with some troubled teens. I think she sought acceptance so eagerly that she gave her attention to anyone who gave her theirs. And Brian and I had no knowledge of any of the students she attended school with, nor their parents, making our guidance minimal. When we did see signs that these particular girls and boys may not be the quality of people we wished for her to hang out with, she became upset when we mentioned it. Realizing that everyone needs to learn the hard way at times, we did our best to support her without completely interfering with her choices. Unfortunately, by the end of her sophomore year, she learned for herself that she had made poor choices in trusting this group of kids.

There was one particular incident where things came to a head, and Brian and I finally had to intervene. We recalled how Abi's specialists, when educating us about her brain injuries, warned us about her inability to see danger and to make good choices as a result. She had difficulty making quick decisions.

Where those of us who have fully functional brains would naturally seem to know right from wrong, Abi could not always decipher between the two. Taking people at their word, Abi was sometimes naive, and, as a result, became an easy target for those with less-than-pure intentions.

She came home one weekend morning after spending the night with these friends, and we immediately knew something was off. Abi was typically a sweet-spirited girl who was eager to please, especially when it came to her family. But this particular day, she had quite an attitude toward us, and the situation escalated as we asked her about her time at her friend's house. Once she calmed down a bit, Brian pulled out information from her that left me as angry as I have ever been with another human. She confirmed our suspicions about this group of teens, telling us that their parents hosted parties for them and their friends. Both boys and girls spent the night at their house, and the girls' mother would make them cocktails, while encouraging them to do "adult" things in her presence.

I won't go into details about everything we learned that morning, but Brian had to stop me from driving to that house to confront the girls' mother. I was angrier than a wet hen! Parents, especially mothers, are supposed to protect children— even teenagers. Knowing that this woman not only allowed but encouraged disgusting things to happen in her presence made me livid. Abigail was 15 years old, and that other mother set her up with an 18-year-old man! Abi had never dated before and didn't know the first thing about dating. In my mind, something had to be done about the mother's recklessness. She should face consequences for such terrible behavior.

After Brian talked me down, I decided I would go to the administration office on Monday and talk to the chaplain at the school. Brian and I told Abigail that she could not hang out with these derelicts anymore, and we kept her on a short leash to make sure she didn't.

When I met with the chaplain, he explained to me that the

teens had a bad reputation, but when he saw Abi hanging around them at school, he assumed she was just like them. "Birds of a feather," right? He didn't know us at all, and that's why we always talk to our kids about the importance of surrounding yourself with those who are known for the good things they do and say. But it still was unsettling to me that nobody thought of warning us as the newbies in the school about these and other potential dangers.

After the mother who instigated these bad behaviors heard that I would no longer allow Abi to go to their home, she took matters into her own hands and began to bully Abi at school. She somehow thought it was appropriate to confront Abi several times just to tell her how disappointed she was that Abigail "squealed" on her. Abi was frightened, and all the kids who hung out in that crowd shunned her. Meanwhile, because she had "flocked" with people of the wrong "feathers," the students who were good role models wanted nothing to do with her.

Being a social butterfly myself and having a great network of friends, I longed for her to have girlfriends to hang out and be teenagers with—but the "right kind" of kids. It was terribly unfortunate, and my heart broke for her.

That was just one example of how her brain injury created some uncomfortable situations for Abi as she grew up. I am certain that she didn't feel good about herself when she made those choices but wanted so badly to be accepted that she was willing to compromise her values. Don't get me wrong, most of us do this from time to time as we grow and struggle with who we are and who we are meant to be, but Abi seemed so much more vulnerable at every stage of childhood and adolescence because of the parts of her brain that were damaged beyond repair.

Abi and the Notre Dame Swim Team

Abi's involvement with the swim team proved to be the best thing that could have happened to her high school experience. I am so grateful for her incredible coaches and teammates, who, after she struggled to find her place during her sophomore year, embraced her as one of their own. Knowing that her dad was a star swimmer in high school (and still holds the record for the 4x100 freestyle relay over 30 years later), Abi made the brave decision to "dive" into the team in the fall of her junior year.

I couldn't believe it when she told us that she was trying out for the team since she had never swum competitively. Brian and I both beamed with pride as we reflected upon a time when her left side wouldn't allow her to swim in a straight line. When she was a little tyke, we called her Nemo after the fish in the Disney movie *Finding Nemo.* So, to see her excited—and honestly, nervous, let's be honest— about giving her dad's favorite sport a shot was neat.

The girls on the team were extraordinarily disciplined and kept themselves out of trouble, which was a stark contrast to the friends that I spoke of earlier. They guided her as the newbie and cheered for her from the sidelines as she swam each event. Electric energy was always in the air at the meets, and there was never drama between the teammates or between the opposing teams. Brian and I looked forward to watching these talented young ladies and volunteering at all the home meets. I had never experienced anything so exhilarating as a parent, except for the years that I spent as a band mom while Noah was in the marching band and drumline.

At the beginning of that first season, Abi was still a new swimmer and primarily swam the 50-yard and 100-yard freestyle (or "free" in swimmer's terms) and backstroke events. As she improved her techniques, she took on more events like breaststroke (or "breast"). She even went far out of her comfort zone and pushed herself to swim the 500 free once! That was incredible to watch because we knew it took serious courage and conditioning to swim that event. But she wanted to do it, so do it she did!

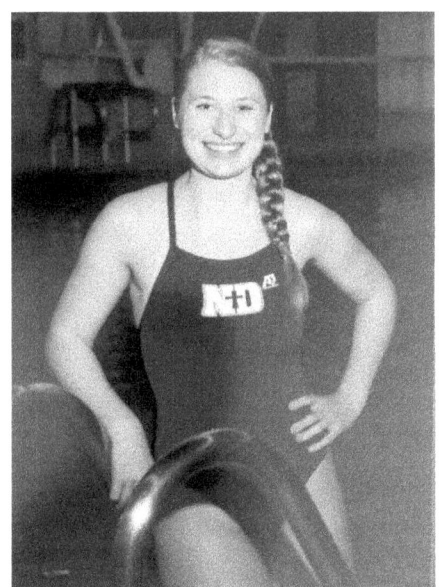

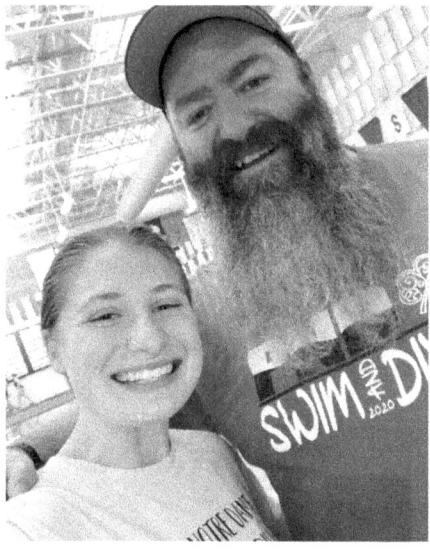

Abi and her swim coach

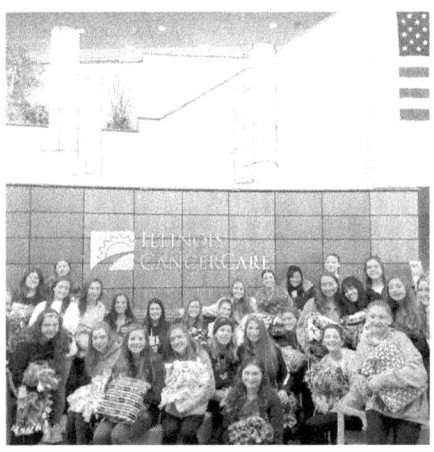

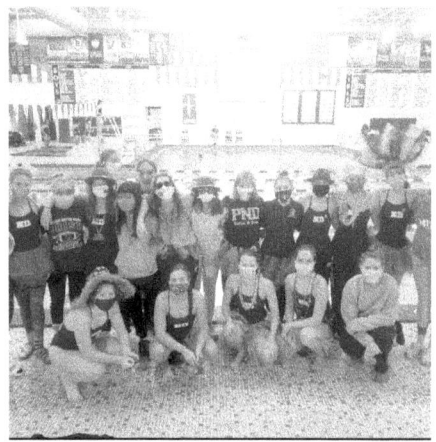

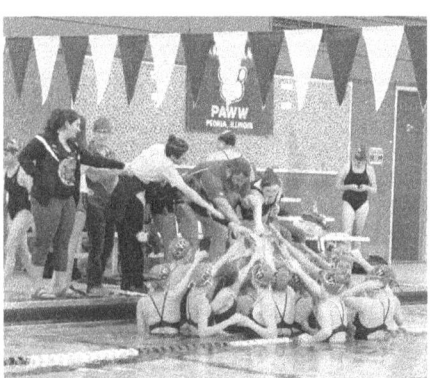

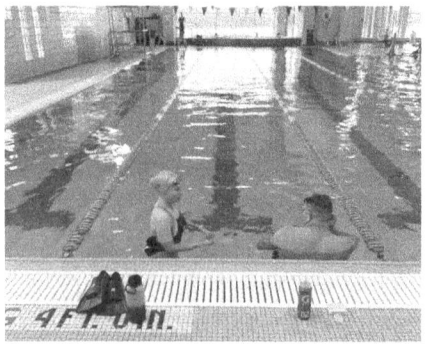

Abi and Brian practicing swim together

Annually, the team made tie blankets, a fun team-building experience that provided warmth for those receiving cancer treatments at Illinois Cancer Care in Peoria. The girls hand-picked fabrics that paired with each patient's interests, shopped together for their supplies at the local fabric store, and created each blanket at the school library. Abi's favorite part of this experience was delivering their creations to the patients individually and learning their stories. She has a fond memory of the man for whom she made a Chicago Bears blanket who told her he had been receiving treatments for a number of years. She was struck by how young he appeared and the conversation she had with him left a lasting impression on her.

Abi the Volunteer

Abi's heart was much larger and softer than the typical young person, and she enjoyed helping others whenever she could, seeking out opportunities on her own. Part of the graduation requirements for all students was to clock a number of volunteer hours. During one of the summers while I was volunteering for a local soup kitchen, Abigail joined me once a week to either work in the kitchen or at the window serving clients. It warmed my mama heart to serve our community together in such a way, knowing that many people might have gone without food otherwise.

Since feeding those in need is one of my all-time favorite ways to give back, Abi also volunteered with me at a local food bank, where we boxed up food to ship to those in need, and at a men's Christian rescue ministry in the kitchen. She also joined her bestie volunteering at a Catholic church fish fry during lent for two years. And since she knows all too well what it means to be a sickly child, she developed an interest in St. Jude and volunteered for race-day registration one year.

Volunteerism is still as important to her as ever, and she has carried this passion into her college days. She now volunteers for Best Buddies as a buddy to a disabled young lady her age.

Given Abi's interest in special education, it was no surprise to me that she wanted to help a peer in need of special attention, and it made me so proud to see her get excited about spending time with her buddy.

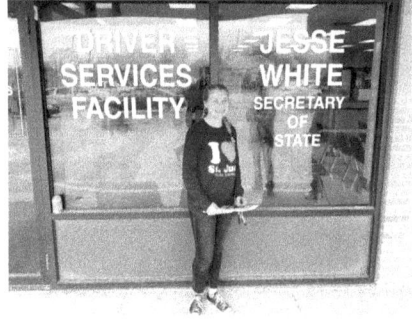

Abi gets her driver's license

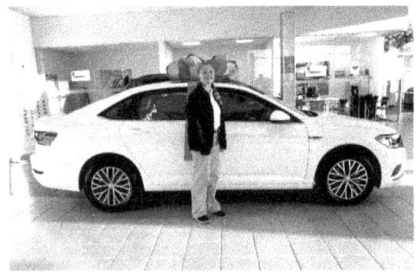

Abi with her first car

Getting Her Driver's License

Abi's coursework was becoming increasingly difficult, and when she got behind the wheel of a car in driver's education, our worries as parents again went into overdrive. Given her history with seizure activity, Abi needed clearance from her doctors to climb behind the wheel, which will forever be required each time she needs to renew her driver's license. Although she had been seizure-free for nine years by the time she started driving, I couldn't shake the nagging fear that she could still have one while driving. It was difficult for me to rest anytime she drove, especially after she became a fully licensed driver and was in her car alone. But those fears come with the territory no matter who we are and what our children have experienced.

Abi became the proud owner of a Volkswagen Jetta on October 11, 2018, just a few days before she turned 16, and was able to practice driving it while she had her permit. Teaching Noah to drive was stressful enough and he had no real inhibitions or disabilities, so imagine how strung out I was while sitting in the passenger seat with Abi and her permit. While Noah was a typical teen boy and thought he knew everything about everything, Abi was the polar opposite. She was timid behind the wheel and emotional at times. I was on edge while she drove, cautious not to grip the passenger side door handle for dear life, slam on my imaginary brake, or make noises when all I wanted to do was scream. If I were to do any of these things, she would freak out. Suffice it to say that Brian would end up taking these duties over for me.

Abi was a bit behind getting her license because neither she nor Brian nor I wanted to proceed until she was fully prepared. But on April 18, 2019, Abi finally became a licensed driver. Extremely cautious (sometimes to a fault), she drove to and from school each day, and when she got her first job almost two months later, she drove back and forth to work. Other than that, she didn't drive much at first since she still lacked confidence in her driving abilities.

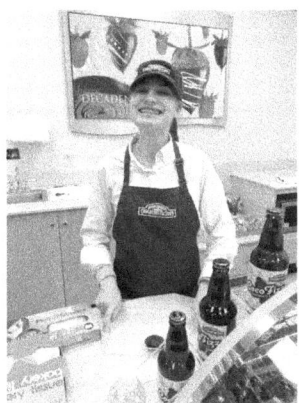

Abi at her first job

While traveling to gas up before a swim banquet, Abi totaled her Jetta. She was stopped in traffic, waiting to make a left turn (sound familiar?) into the gas station parking lot. Misjudging the distance between her car and the one approaching from the opposite direction, she was struck by the driver, who couldn't slow down in time. The accident was her fault, and the county sheriff's deputy issued her a

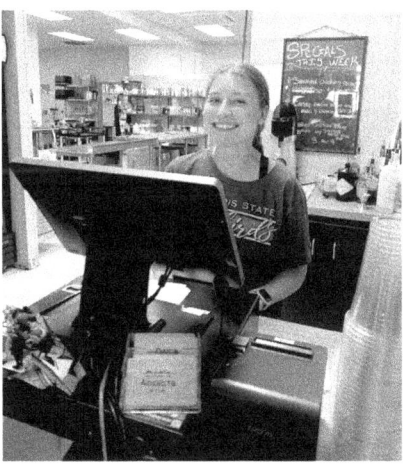

Abi working at her second job

ticket after investigating the scene. Thankfully, besides some very large bruises on her legs, she was virtually unharmed. But after viewing the camera footage from inside the gas station, the deputy told us that, with the collision being head-on, she could have easily been killed had she not been driving a Volkswagen with full driver-side air bag deployment. You better believe we bought her another Volkswagen after hearing that! While Brian and I took care of the final report with the deputy, Abigail called Noah to come and get her so that she wouldn't miss her banquet, and off she went. She was very lucky that day.

Not long after the Jetta was totaled and she became the proud owner of a Tiguan, she again struck another vehicle on her way to school. Thankfully, it was a minor fender bender, and nobody was hurt. She was quite shaken by her driving abilities after that— and to be quite frank, so was I! She took time away from the wheel for a bit until she was ready to give it another go and has been accident-free since, thank God. I still cannot relax when I know she is driving on the highway, and I track her on my phone until I know she is home safely.

My PTSD Conquers Me

While Abi was taking time away from driving, my PTSD went into full swing at the most inopportune time. Abigail and I took a day trip to visit one of my high school girlfriends and her family who lived about an hour and a half away. Until that day, I had never had any problem driving on the highway, which was remarkable, all things considered. I drove us to my friend's place where we had a fun pool day, and as night fell, we began the drive back to Peoria.

After being on the road for only 20 minutes or so, I experienced a panic attack while driving. My vehicle even sensed that I was having a moment because it started chirping at me and displayed on my dash a message to take a break, which really freaked me out. I was shaking uncontrollably, and my heart was racing out of my chest.

There were almost nothing but semitrucks that late at night, making me nervous, and I asked Abigail if she could drive the rest of the way home. Nope, not a chance! She was panicking too, and I pulled off the highway at the nearest exit and did what all independent, liberated women do—I called my husband to save me. He settled me down enough to try to drive again with an alternate way back. Thanks to GPS, I found my way home using back roads after I calmed down enough to climb back behind the wheel, but I was terrified.

Since that night, I have not been able to drive on the highway. I have tried unsuccessfully to win this battle inside my brain and have sought the help of therapy to at least make sense of it. Even after all that happened in 2002, I never hesitated to drive on freeways surrounded by vehicles of all sizes, but something triggered my worst fears that night and I cannot seem to get past it. My therapist explained that I had been in survival mode and did what I had to do when the kids needed me to drive them. There must have been something about the timing of both kiddos being able to drive themselves that caused my "flight" mode to overpower my "fight" mode.

Whatever the reason, after 16 years of experiencing zero issues behind the steering wheel, my independence and the freedom that came from the ability to drive anywhere at any time was suddenly gone. But remember what I said about adapting and survival of the fittest? I am still able to get from one town to another in my own way and on my own terms using back roads and the navigation app on my phone. Granted, it might take me twice as long, but where there's a will, there's a way. Gotta love technology and a person's will to carry on!

Noah's Journey

Noah graduated high school in May 2018, and with dreams of attending the University of Missouri (Mizzou) in Columbia— where we would have to pay out-of-state tuition—he decided to join the Air National Guard instead. This was about the time that my mom fell quite ill with her own battle with cancer. That summer and fall were a bit of an emotional blur. On one hand, we had incredible highs, watching our son graduate with honors and enlist to follow his dad's footsteps to become part of our United States military, and on the other, I was plagued with the pain of driving back and forth to be with a cancer-riddled parent.

While Noah waited for a spot to open up at Air Force basic training and technical school, he attended our local community college and continued to live with us. For a new high school graduate who was ready to leave Peoria in his rearview mirror, it had been tough, especially since his friends had spread themselves all over the US for a more traditional college experience. When the day came for him to leave the nest, he did so with mixed emotions.

On November 13, 2019, after waiting a full year for his orders, Noah left us all crying our eyes out in the Peoria airport to leave for basic training in San Antonio, Texas. When I looked into his baby blues for the last time, I could see that he was both excited for the next chapter to begin and scared of the unknown. We had no contact with him while he was away, except for a quick, unexpected FaceTime call on Thanksgiving that made my mama heart sing.

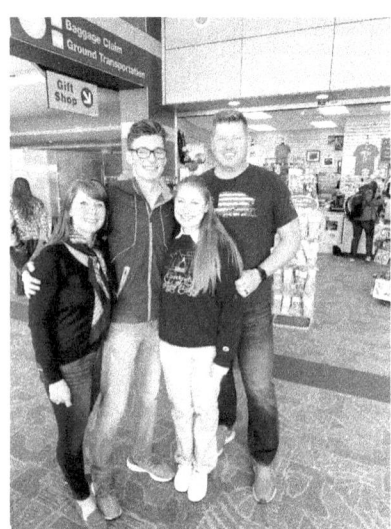 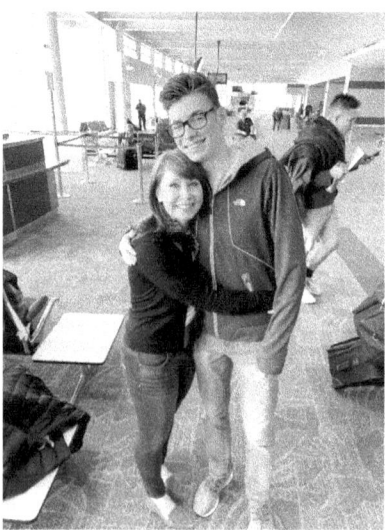

Seeing Noah off at the airport

It was sad for the three of us left behind, and we were forced to find a new normal—thankfully, a concept we were not unfamiliar with. We wrote him letters (well, I wrote letters while the other two sat and watched) and looked forward to seeing him at his graduation in January 2020. Until that day, we would carry around our "Flat Noah"—a paint stir stick with a photo of his face laminated and taped to it—with us everywhere we went. It became a fun time for all of our friends too, as we would pose with "Flat Noah" for photos during the plethora of holiday events we attended. I love looking back on all those photos when we were doing what we could to lighten the mood—something that was always important to us when we encountered heartache.

Noah Graduates from Basic Training

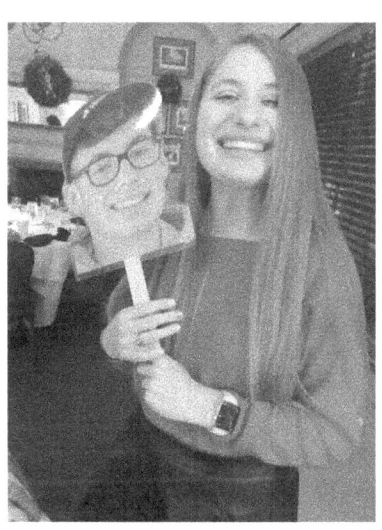

Abi with Flat Noah

In January 2020, we headed to San Antonio where we would have the honor and privilege of witnessing Noah's graduation from the US Air Force Basic Training. Tammy, Doug, and Alyssa flew in as well, and we all stayed in an Airbnb not far from base. What a magical time it was! When I first put my eyes on the freshly-buzzed head of my firstborn on January 9, my heart felt like it had burst inside my chest. Noah had advanced to a leadership position in his unit, and as the graduates ran out into the arena where their loved ones waited, I spotted him in the front of the pack, next to his fellow airman who was carrying the American flag. At that moment, the dam that had previously held back my tears ripped wide open. It's not often during our lifetime that we can experience such an intense feeling of pride, and Brian and I both beamed with it.

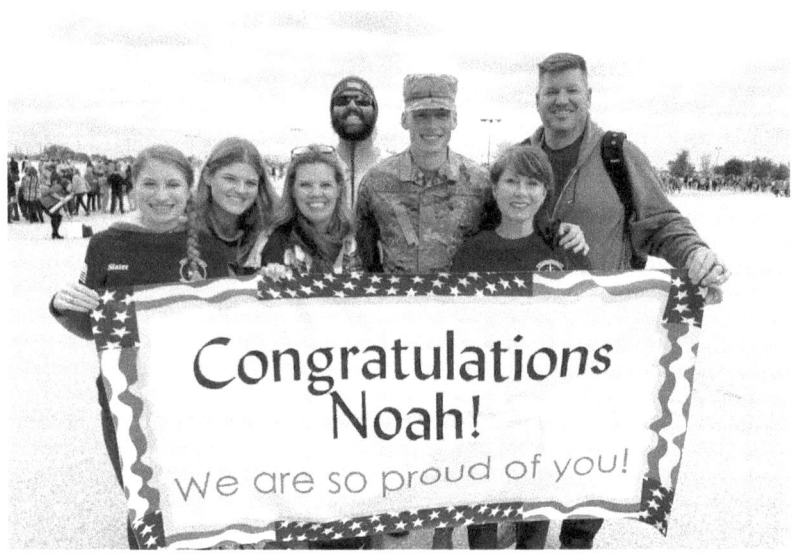

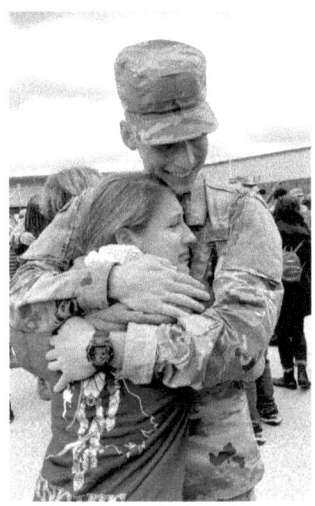

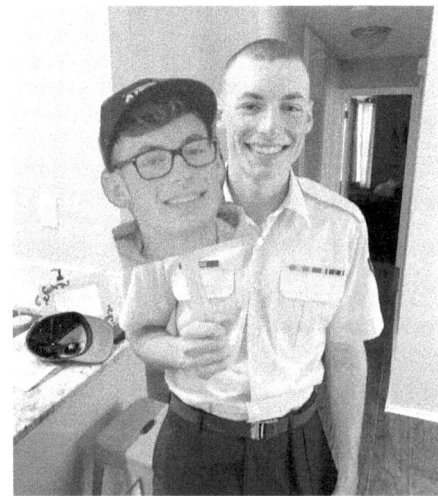

After their initial run through the stadium, we, along with hundreds of other proud parents and loved ones, went through the torture of waiting for our young men and women to get cleaned up and into their fatigues. When the moment we had all anticipated with such incredible joy arrived, and we were allowed to wander in search of our uniformed troops, the six of us hastily searched the crowd of camo until we found Noah. In the sea of emotional people, I locked eyes on my guy and touched him on the shoulder, and we were finally able to hug each other. Abi and I cried rivers of tears after not having communicated for months with him. After all the hugging was temporarily out of our systems, and the tears were replaced with perma-smiles, we were allowed to wander the base and tour their barracks, which was quite cool.

We spent the weekend off and on base, taking every opportunity we could to explore the city of San Antonio with our new airman. Each day there were different events for the airmen and their loved ones to experience, along with the graduation and formal ceremonies taking place on January 10. It was awesome to get the chance to meet many of the friends he made at training. Noah was extremely preoccupied and emotional much of the time that we spent together, turning many of our happy moments into those full of anxiety, as we knew our time together was short and he would soon head to technical school. We did our best to make the most of our time until we dropped him off at base and watched him walk away and board the bus to Gulfport, Mississippi. Our hearts were shattered all over again, knowing it would be many months before we would see him again.

College Bound

As Abigail plugged away at high school classes, extracurriculars like swimming, choir, school dances, and hanging out with the few friends that she had, she gave a lot of thought to what she wanted to do after graduation. She was always impressed by a couple of her teachers who had really made a difference in her school experience, including her pre-K, first-grade teacher, and fourth-grade teacher. These ladies had taken extra time to get to know Abigail and advocated for her to the best of their abilities—it left a positive impression on Abi. So when she spoke about what she might like to do in terms of work after college, she often talked about being a teacher.

She applied to a college in a city not far from Peoria known for its education programs, and upon acceptance, she made the decision to major in elementary education, specializing in special education. It made my heart melt when she told me that she wanted to do for others what her teachers had done for her. Teachers really can make such a difference in students' lives, and I'm not sure they are aware of just how much of a difference is made. I commend all teachers for what they do.

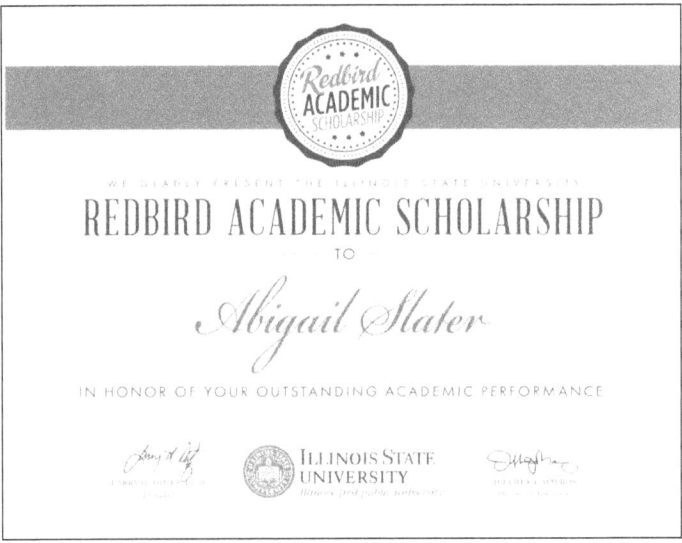

Abigail's senior year was one filled with mostly positive emotions, and great strides were made in her independence and grades. By this time, she had grown into a force to be reckoned with. She was organized and kept ahead of all her coursework deadlines, successfully juggling her academic world with her personal world. Although her high school career at the private Catholic school got off to a rocky start, she now was confident enough in herself and what she brought to the table that she stayed away from the troublemakers, even if it meant she stood alone. She held down a part-time job as well, increasing her self-confidence and feeding her love of money. It was funny to see how two children born of the same parents could be entirely different from one another: Abi loved to count her money and save it, while Noah blew it faster than he could earn it. He always had various part-time jobs throughout high school as well, but never seemed to have any money. We laugh about their differences to this day.

As the end of her high school career approached, Abi attended her senior prom with one of her girlfriends, and there was no agenda for after-prom partying or any other devious things teenagers do (we were thankful for that indeed!). They had a wonderful time and looked absolutely beautiful and carefree. We probably took about 250 photos around Peoria before sending them on their way to the dance. Abi was delighted that day, and my heart was full.

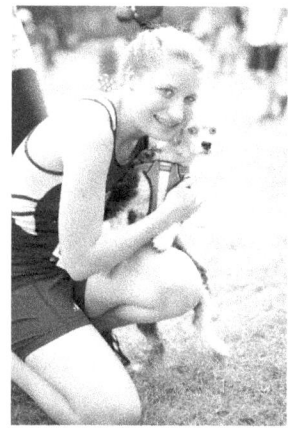

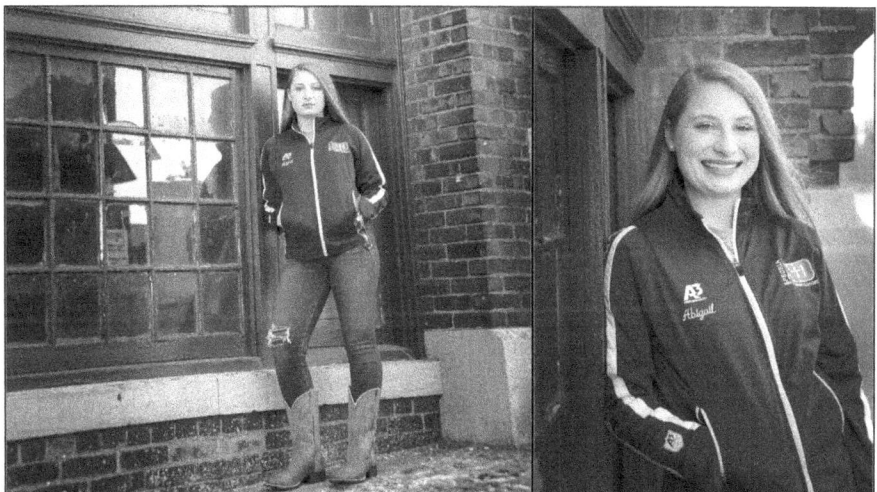

Graduation occurred on May 30, 2021, with Abi's party the following weekend. She had finally done it! After all the hard work, tears, frustration, peaks, valleys, medicines, hospitalizations, and learning experiences, Abigail was a high school graduate with a college acceptance letter in her hands. She enjoyed the fruits of her labor for the summer, while planning to attend Illinois State University, home of the Redbirds. What an accomplishment for a girl who was never expected to live a "normal" life! Her life was anything but normal, it was extraordinary, a testament to what God is capable of.

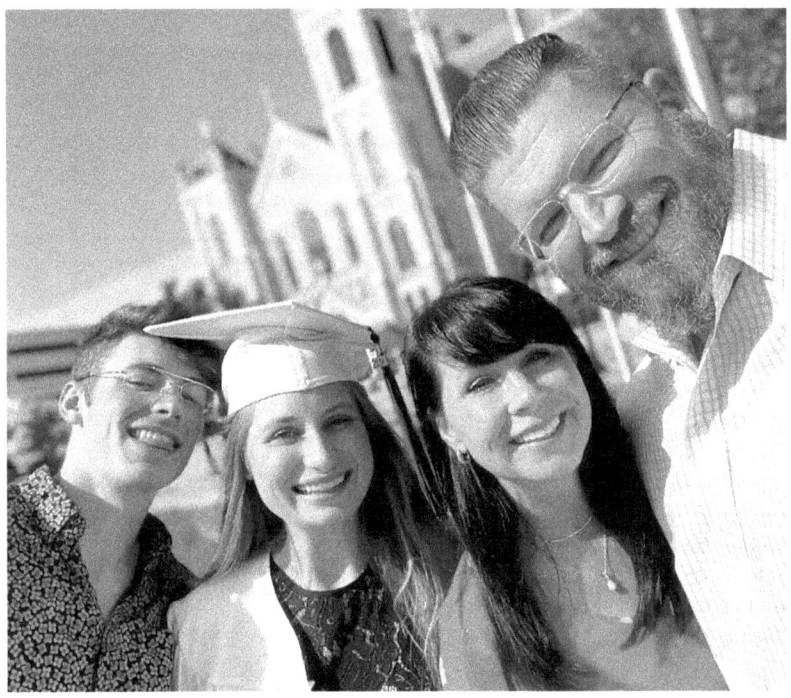

Abi's high school graduation day

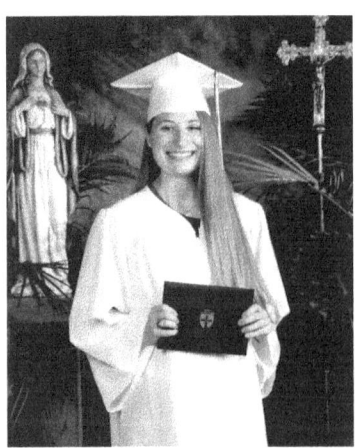
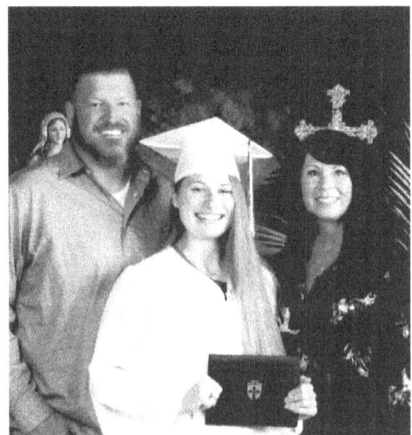

We moved Abi into a dorm her freshman year, and she became acquainted with the campus before classes began so she would feel prepared for her first day. Abi was always extremely organized because it helped to ease her anxiety about the unknown, and she took great pleasure in buying planners where she would color-code her classes and assignments with pens and highlighters in all the colors of the rainbow. She communicated with all her professors before each semester began to familiarize them with her accommodations, and never hesitated to ask questions and visit them during their office hours. Taking to heart what her military father always told our kids, "If you are early, you're on time and if you are on time, you're late," Abi has always been the early bird.

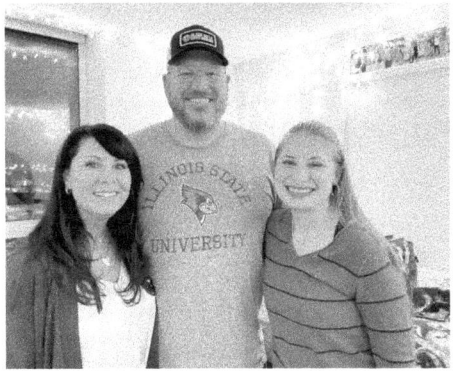 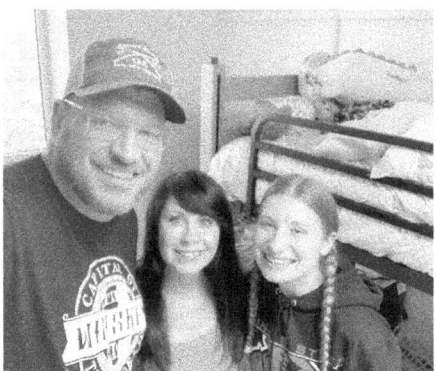

Moving Abi into the dorms

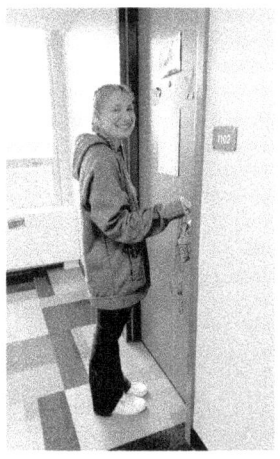

The funny thing about college for Abigail was that something just seemed to click right away. Since she was always such a hard worker, it was no surprise that she could be incredibly independent away from home. Like any parent of a college-bound student, I was nervous about her being away from home but took comfort in the fact that she was just a 45-minute drive away from our house. I would see her often throughout her college years, but the day we moved her onto campus was an emotional day for us all, and I cried both tears of sorrow and joy all the way home.

COVID

As is typical for students who live with roommates for the first time in their lives, Abi struggled in the dorms with her first roommate, and then with her second one. There were some large cultural differences with her first roommate, and due to it being a heavy COVID year, rules for managing the disease were rigid. Masks had to be worn at all times on campus, including in the dorm rooms, and the school officials weren't fond of students leaving campus. (Plus, we were unsure how COVID would affect Abi if she were to catch it.) Her roommate was nonchalant about the mask rules and was rarely ever in their dorm room because she liked to party off-campus with her friends, which was normal for college students. But given the circumstances of the world at that time, she put others at risk and ended up testing positive for COVID.

The protocol for the university included quarantining students who tested positive for COVID, which was close to half of them by the time the school year was over. But because Abi lived closer to home than her roommate did, and the quarantine rooms were full, Abi was asked by the college administration to move home for two weeks. So, donning our masks, we picked her up outside the dorm and loaded her things into the bed of the truck. When she entered the backseat, she reeked of pot, which led to many questions for the ride home. It turns out that so many of the students living in the dorm at that time smoked pot that it was virtually impossible for the resident assistants (RAs) to stop it.

This happened twice while she lived in the dorms. When her freshman year was over, Abi made the decision to get her own apartment. After the first semester with the partier from Chicago, Abi asked to get a new roommate. At the beginning of her second semester, we moved her into the room right next door. Awkward! And while her new roommate was a friend that Abi had made during her first semester, she didn't have the best experience living with her either. The girls were different in their study habits and kept different schedules. It became a teaching moment through which Abi learned she was better off on her own. The girls would try to remain friends, but the large campus and different fields of study created an environment where it proved to be more work than either was ready to put forth.

Chasing the Honor Roll and More Growth in College

While Abi was never a high achiever in terms of grades in high school, she excelled in college. Maybe it was because she found her passion as a special education student, or maybe it had more to do with her general growth into a woman on a mission, but something really clicked in her that propelled her forward. I watched her develop a deep love for school in general, but for the first time in her life, as a college student, she enjoyed learning. One of her favorite pastimes is reading. After all the effort she put forth in RTI as a young child, it is more satisfying than I could ever describe in words to witness her love for reading books. She even recommends books to me that she thinks I will like, and I forage through the library in her bedroom while she is at school, looking for a new gem to dive into.

Her sophomore year at ISU gave her an amazing opportunity to present something of great value to her Intro to Special Education class. Seeing a need to educate her fellow students on epilepsy, she approached her teacher with the idea of giving a 30-minute presentation about the basics of seizures. Her teacher happily scheduled the time for Abigail to present during class time, and she went to work right away. The presentation included defining epilepsy and its causes, as well as seizure first aid, especially as it applies to the classroom. What I found spectacular was that after her talk was over, one of Abi's class-mates told her that she too had epilepsy and commended Abi on the information she provided to everyone. What a remarkable way to, yet again, make something positive from a less-than-desirable experience.

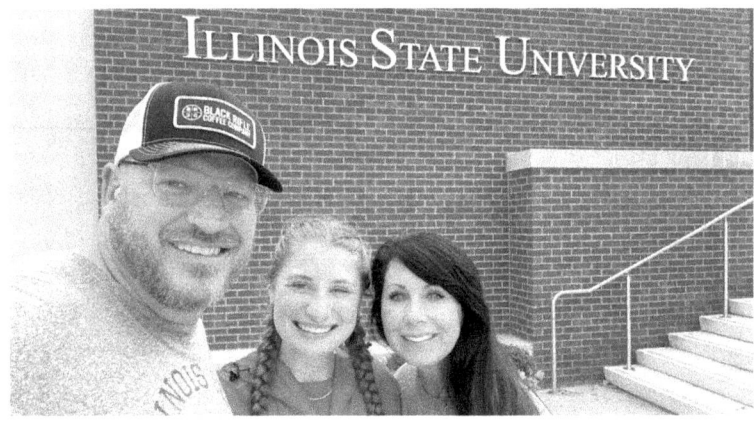

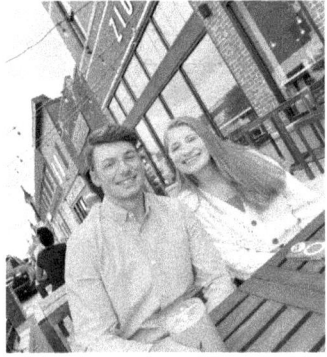
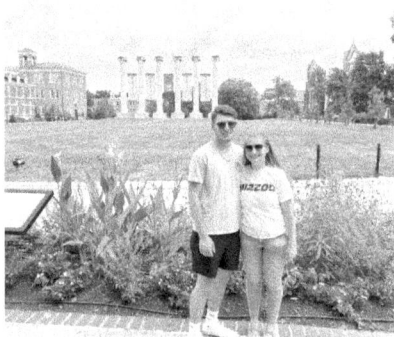

Routine Medical Follow-Ups

During the summers, Abi visits her specialists for routine checkups while she is home for break and still has MRIs, CT scans, and what is called "shunt series" X-rays, which is an x-ray that shows the entire shunt from the portion that is in her ventricle, all the way down to the abdomen where the shunt tubing ends. She has not had a shunt malfunction since she was released from Children's Hospital of Omaha in 2003, and there has thankfully never been a need for a shunt revision. We feel blessed that things finally seem to have worked themselves out for her and she doesn't have to worry as much about her health as she grows into a young adult, though we all remain cautious in our optimism and are prepared for whatever life may throw her way in terms of physical health.

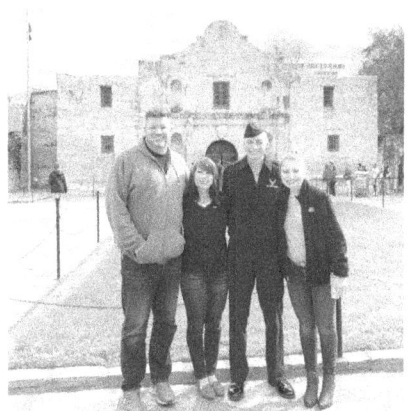

Our family visiting the Alamo after Noah's basic training graduation

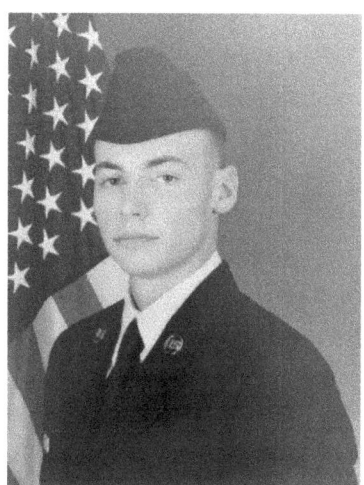

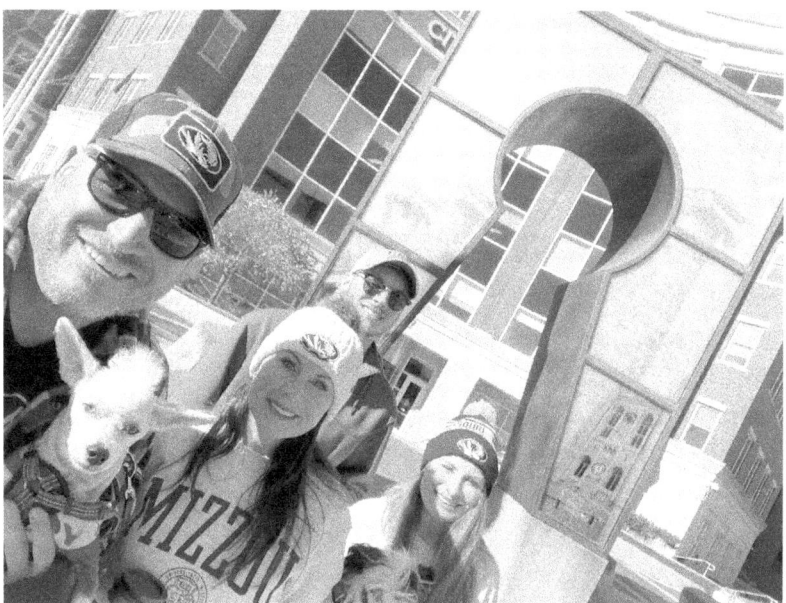

Visiting Noah at Mizzou

The Beginning of a Bright Future

Abi has had a successful college career so far. Remember when her doctors warned us that she would likely never live on her own? On August 11, 2022, we moved her into her first apartment where—you guessed it—she lives on her own. No roommates and nobody to help her navigate her days. Then we moved Noah into another apartment in Columbia—those were certainly busy times! Where she struggled in high school, Abi excelled in college, and she has maintained a 3.5 GPA leading up to her senior year. She even made the dean's list and represented the College of Education at ISU during her last semester of her junior year with a 3.81 GPA, proving that hard work does pay off.

As I wrap up the final chapter to this book, it's the summer before Abi heads into her senior year of college and is preparing to student teach next year in a nearby town. Noah is finishing up his first six-year commitment to the Missouri Air National Guard and is a senior at Mizzou. I have a clear reflection upon the past 20+ years of motherhood, and although the future is much less clear, I am more prepared than I ever was before. God continues to show Himself to me and to my loved ones every day. I have learned that I am much stronger than I know, and it is only because I trust Him to deliver me from all evil, just as He promises in His Word.

Rocking the Empty Nest

While I was initially quite melancholy about both kids flying the coop, it didn't take long for Brian and me to find our footing in this new chapter. The anticipation of no longer having the kids around was worse than the reality, and I took hold of the opportunity with both hands and a firm grip to do all the work I had previously put off. For the previous 20-plus years, I put my husband and children at the front of the line in all that I did, and now it was finally time for me to explore who I was and what I wanted to make of the second half of my life (God willing). But what did that mean? Like a blank canvas to a painter, I first needed to become inspired to not just start, but to create something beautiful.

In March 2015, Brian and I went into business for ourselves once again, after we had both been working in the financial industry for a large company. He had been an advisor since we left Nebraska (minus the few years that we operated our flooring and concrete business), and I had been working as an on-call assistant to advisors at different locations in the Peoria area for a few years. Realizing just how limited he had become with what he could offer his clients in his position then, we both decided after months of deliberation and exploration that we would become independent advisors with a new broker-dealer.

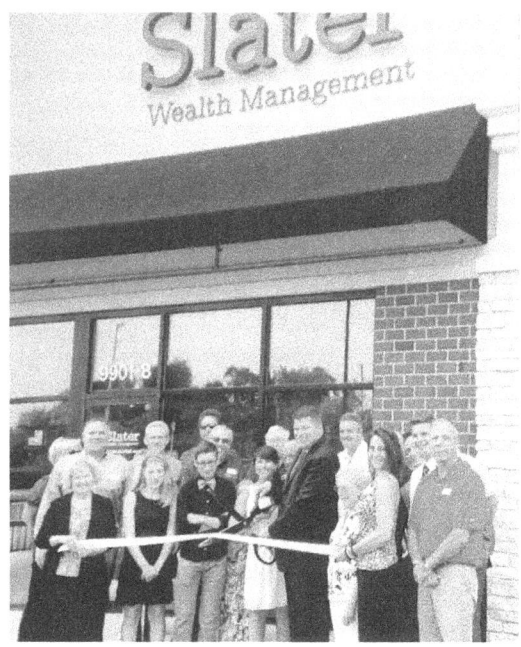

Ribbon cutting ceremony for our new business

We plowed away at turning this idea into reality and we have been building our business since, with much success. I function as the operations manager for Slater Wealth Management and Brian is the main financial advisor, earning an invitation each year to our broker-dealer's annual conference. After being behind the scenes for seven years, assisting him and the other advisors who had come and gone, I decided to study for and take my licensing exams, which was no small feat. Those exams were the toughest I have ever sat for, but I passed them and now hold my Series 7 and 66 registrations, becoming a registered assistant. This means that I have many of the same registrations as Brian with the Financial Industry Regulatory Authority (FINRA).

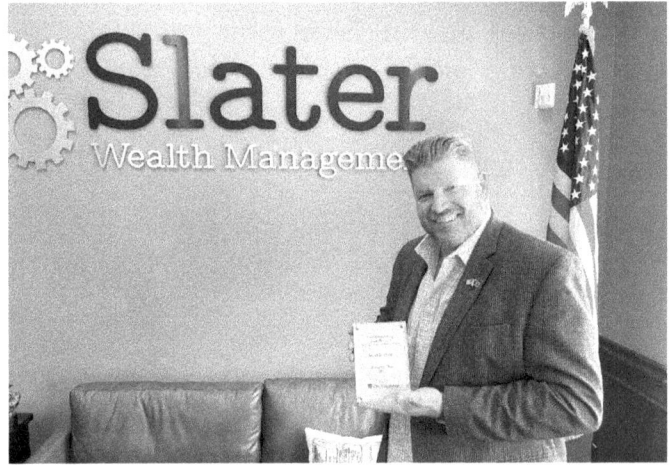

Brian receiving one of his many production awards

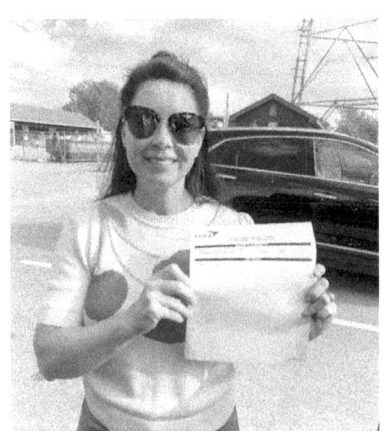
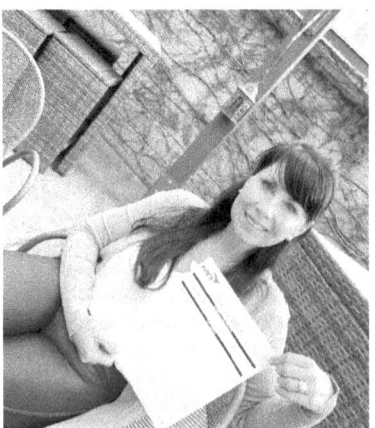

Me after passing my series 66 and 7 licensing exams

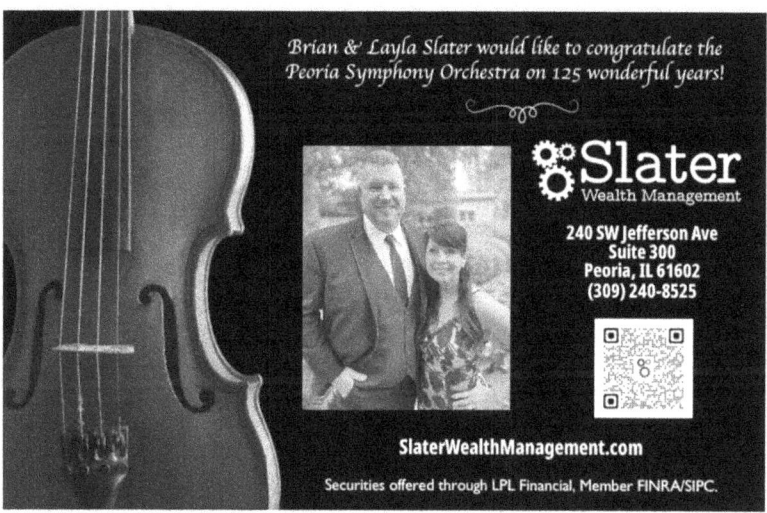

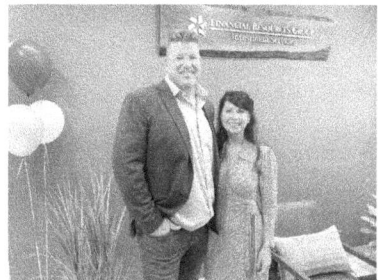

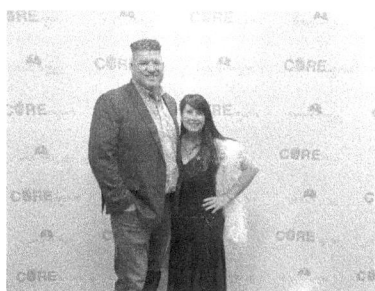

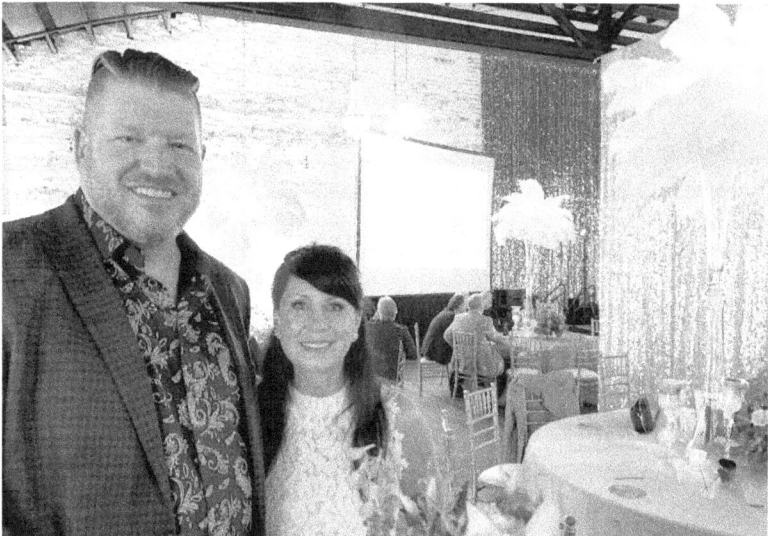

Brian and me at various fundraisers

Since Brian and I are rocking this empty nest that we have created, we have both been able to spread our wings and experience new things. Our small business is thriving, and we both enjoy serving our community in various capacities. I believe that if you are unwilling to take the necessary steps to change what is not working for you or your community, you have no right to complain about your situation. I am doing my best to work for the greater good and to never bring forth a complaint without also bringing a solution. Brian and I both sit on executive boards for local nonprofit organizations, and I serve in a number of professional organizations. Because I am passionate about politics, especially on a local level, I am honored to participate as an election judge and support my party in volunteer efforts. Since entertaining and throwing parties is a pastime I have always enjoyed, I spend a great deal of time on planning committees for fundraising events. I keep myself busy learning new creative skills by taking various art classes at our local art guild. Oh, and I decided to write a book!

One of our favorite pastimes, both as small business owners and as compassionate Peorians, is to sponsor and attend fundraising events for some of our favorite local nonprofits. Whether it's a golf outing to raise money for the Blue Star Mothers, a gala that benefits the Family House of Peoria, or a luncheon that supports the local crisis nursery, odds are you'll find Brian or me there. If we cannot attend, we likely sponsor on some level.

Our network of friends is vast and diverse, and since we lack a real extended family unit, our friends have become our family. The historic neighborhood where we now reside is lively with activities and gatherings of all kinds, keeping us quite busy in our own pod of Peoria. The street is filled with artists from all over the country, musicians, businesspeople, politicians, doctors, lawyers, and a plethora of other occupations, which maintains a level of diversity and interesting conversations. Our great friends from our old school district even moved to our new street after we moved, putting the icing on the cake.

We travel as often as the business will allow, either as a couple, a family, or with our closest friends, and have discovered a great deal of the world I never imagined I would see. With a long list of places I still want to visit, we have plans to travel much more as time and finances allow. Creating professional and personal goals keeps me motivated to continue to work hard. I believe in balancing work and fun to live a rich life, and I encourage everyone to do the same.

My body has healed as much as can be expected given the extent of my injuries, although I struggle from time to time with the aftermath of broken bones and tissue tears that will never mend themselves completely. Thankfully, I have all the right specialists (like my wonderful chiropractor, massage therapist, and primary care physician) to keep me ahead of the aging curve as much as possible. The PTSD will likely linger, but you will never see me give into it; I will always fight it with all I have, and because of that attitude, I am taking small but mighty steps toward driving on the highway again. Until the day my fear of big trucks traveling at high speeds subsides, I continue to find beauty in the back roads and have even convinced my husband to occasionally do the same.

Beauty in the Back Roads

With Abigail living about 40 miles away from us, we visit her at school often, and when I drive myself, I take a two-lane highway to avoid the increasingly fast traffic of the freeway. I thoroughly enjoy my time alone, driving through small towns and reminiscing about the one in which I was raised, while Brian's mission is always to get there in the least amount of time legally possible. But one of my fondest memories of our travels together is a time last year when I convinced him to drive the back roads in my tiny, aged convertible with me, stopping along the way at my favorite small-town coffee shop.

Enjoying the breezy autumn day and the conversations we had, with some of our favorite tunes in the background, was a highlight for me. The clouds hung in the deep blue sky like cotton balls, and as we drank our coffee, I watched the corn tassels dance in the breeze from the passenger side.

After we visited with Abi and began to head back home, Brian asked me, "Back roads or highway?" to which I replied, "It's your call. I appreciate you humoring me on the way here." Fully expecting him to take the highway home, I climbed into my midlife-crisis red Mini Cooper and was tickled pink when he didn't take the exit that would take us home via interstate traffic. I looked at him with the biggest smile on my face and he said, "I actually kind of like the back roads." That's love, folks—that right there is what adaptation, empty nesting, and compromise looks like.

On the way home with the top down, it began to rain, but hey, that's life, right? There will always be blue skies and sunshine, mixed with stormy weather (but hopefully no more crashes). It's what you decide to do with those darker moments that define you and the life that you choose. Typical of our light-hearted nature, we enjoyed the frigid drops for a few moments before we decided to pull over and put the top back up while we laughed and made plans for our next back-road adventure.

Acknowledgments

I would like to thank the following people for all they did to transform my idea of writing my story into the book that you now hold in your hands.

Brian, I cannot even begin to shed light with words on how much I love you. You are the rock upon which this family is built and your love and encouragement means more to me than I could ever show. I am certain that, without you holding us all together through Abi's early years, we would never have come out of the wreckage with so few scars.

Abigail, I am amazed by you every single day and admire your ability to "just keep swimming," even when you want nothing more than to give up. Your sweet spirit is unmatched, your never ending smile lights up even the darkest situations, and your willingness to always see the good in people is inspiring. You are one of the brightest lights in my life and you make me want to be the best human I can be.

Noah, thank you for being flexible as a little tyke while your sister's needs took precedence over all things and for being such a loving big brother to her. She adores you more than you will likely ever know. You are now and always will be my "sunshine."

Of course I need to thank my mom and dad for all they did for me. The home they made for us was one of love, honesty, integrity, accountability, and discipline. I owe them much of my success for teaching me the importance of independence and hard work.

I want to thank Stephanie, Brandy, Amy, Brian, Abi,

Kathryn, Bonnie, Ivette, and Becky for your input as I wrote this book. Your time and energy were much appreciated.

Thanks to all who played a part in my rescue on that fateful day, the medical personnel at Saunders County Hospital, Bryan LGH, St. Elizabeth Hospital, and Children's Hospital of Omaha.

To everyone who worked and volunteered at the Rainbow House while we made it our temporary home, your kindness and generosity aided in our recovery just as much as anyone's did. After all these years, I credit you with the work I do now for my local hospitality house.

To my NRCS and NRD coworkers, I don't think I could ever convey how grateful I am to have met you all. My boss Brad, my daily sidekick Marla, Jami, Carol, Joanna, Keith, and many others, were instrumental in my recovery and were my Nebraska family.

The medical staff and OSF Children's Hospital of Illinois who helped us throughout Abi's childhood made an extraordinary difference in a little girl's life who was never expected to accomplish a fraction of what she has already done in her young life. Her pediatrician, Dr. Erickson, who introduced us to early intervention services, and then his predecessor Dr. Ho. Her neurosurgeon, Dr. Lin, neurologists, chiropractic doctor, Dr. Joe Khairallah.

Thank you to Abi's therapists —PT, OT, DT. Medical personnel at the Cleveland Clinic, especially, Dr. Wylie,

Lastly, and most importantly, I thank God. Thank you Lord for loving me, forgiving me, and guiding me through each day since I accepted you into my heart. Thank you for sparing my life and the life of my baby girl so that we can help others. I hope that I accomplish all that you have planned for me in this beautiful life that I was allowed to continue.

About the Author

Born and raised in Monmouth, Illinois, this small-town girl with big dreams shattered expectations by becoming the first in her family to attend college. Layla pursued her bachelor of science degree at Western Illinois University, where she met the man who would eventually become her husband and life partner. Layla then earned her graduate credentials from University of Illinois at Springfield, graduating with her master of arts degree in environmental studies just weeks before becoming a mother to her son, Noah.

Layla and her husband Brian, a veteran of the United States Air Force, own and operate their wealth management business in Peoria, Illinois. Layla is heavily involved in community work, volunteering for a variety of nonprofit local and national organizations. As the mother of a child who has benefitted from early intervention and special education services, Layla is an advocate for those who live with developmental delays and learning disabilities.

Organizations with which Layla is affiliated:

- Member of National Association of Women Business Owners (NAWBO) of Central Illinois

- Member of Junior League of Peoria

- Member of Women in Leadership of Central Illinois

- Member of Impact Central Illinois

- Member of Heart of Illinois Blue Star Mothers

- Executive Board Member of Family House of Peoria

- Election Judge of Peoria County Election Commission

- Volunteer with Hydrocephalus Association

- Epilepsy Awareness Ambassador
  for Epilepsy Foundation

Contact Layla at **saving.abigail.grace@gmail.com**
Follow Layla on Facebook at **Layla Slater**
Follow Layla on Instagram at **saving_abigail_grace**
Learn more at **www.SavingAbigailGrace.com**

Glossary

504 plan: A federal law designed to protect the rights of individuals with disabilities in programs and activities. Regulations require a school district to provide a "free appropriate public education" (FAPE) to each qualified student with a disability who is in the school district's jurisdiction, regardless of the nature or severity of the disability. (US Department of Education)

Bilateral posterior interhemispheric hemorrhage (PBSH): A rare type of subdural hemorrhage that can have a poor prognosis. Usually caused by the rupture of veins in the interhemispheric fissure.

Central venous catheter: A long, flexible tube a provider inserts into a vein in the neck, chest, arm or groin. It leads to the vena cava, a large vein that empties into the heart. A CVC helps the body receive drugs, fluids, or blood for emergency or long-term treatment. It also helps with blood draws. Types include PICC lines and ports. (Cleveland Clinic)

Cerebral palsy: A neurological condition that can present as issues with muscle tone, posture, and/or a movement disorder. (Cleveland Clinic)

Chemosis: Swelling of the conjunctiva, the clear membranes covering the whites of the eye and the inside of the eyelids. (Cleveland Clinic)

Chiropractic: Manual manipulation of the spine to support proper alignment of the skeletal system to improve the body's ability to heal itself.

Complex partial seizure disorder: Also known as focal or partial seizures, these seizures start in one part of the brain and spread to other areas.

Developmental therapy: Treatment for children aged birth to three years who have developmental delays or disabilities using their own interests and relationships.

Diurnal enuresis: Involuntary urination during the daytime when a person is past the age of toilet training.

Early intervention: Services that are available to babies and young children with developmental delays and disabilities and their families. May include speech therapy, physical therapy, and other types of services based on the needs of the child and family. (Centers for Disease Control)

Electroencephalogram (EEG): A test that measures electrical activity in the brain. The test uses small metal discs called electrodes that attach to the scalp. Brain cells communicate via electrical impulses, and this activity shows up as wavy lines on an EEG recording. It is one of the main tests to help diagnose epilepsy. (Mayo Clinic)

Encephalomalacia: Softening or loss of brain tissue after cerebral infarction, cerebral ischemia, infection, craniocerebral trauma, or other injury. (Journal of Craniofacial Surgery)

Family and Medical Leave Act (FMLA): Entitles eligible employees of covered employers to take unpaid, job-protected leave for specified family and medical reasons with continuation of group health insurance coverage under the same terms and conditions as if the employee had not taken leave. (Department of Labor)

Foley catheter: An indwelling urinary catheter, which is left in the bladder for extended periods of time.

Fontanelle: A soft spot in a baby's skull where the bones have not yet fused together.

Gliosis with hemosiderin deposit: A consequence of persistent hemorrhage in the subarachnoid area of the brain. Gliosis occurs when the body produces more or larger glial cells in response to a brain injury. Hemosiderin is a yellowish-brown granular pigment that forms when hemoglobin breaks down and deposition of this occurs when this pigment settles in areas of the posterior cerebellum due to gravity.

Hirschsprung's disease: Affecting the large intestine, Hirschsprung's occurs when cells in the intestine do not develop properly, causing pain, swelling, discomfort, and difficulty in passing stools.

Hyaline membrane disease or Respiratory Distress Syndrome (RDS): A common problem in premature babies occurring when there is not enough surfactant, a liquid made by the lungs that keeps the airways (alveoli) open, present in the lungs. It causes babies to need extra oxygen and help with breathing.

Hydrocephalus: A neurological disorder that causes buildup of cerebral spinal fluid (CSF) in the ventricles of the brain. When the ventricles expand from excess fluid, it causes damage to the surrounding brain cells and pressure builds until remedied with placement of a shunt. There is no cure for hydrocephalus.

Individualized Education Plan (IEP): A legal document developed for students with disabilities that identifies needs through evaluations performed by a team of specialists employed by a school district. This team can include physical therapists, occupational therapists, psychologists, special education teachers, social workers, speech and language pathologists, administrators, and the student's parents. Once the needs are identified, a plan is created, consisting of accommodations for the student with goals stated.

Individualized service plan (ISP): The written details of the supports, activities, and resources required for the individual to achieve personal goals. The Individual Service Plan is developed to articulate decisions and agreements made during a person-centered process of planning and information gathering. It is the equivalent of the IEP, but for private schools. (Illinois DHS)

Intraventricular hemorrhage: Bleeding inside and/or around the ventricles of the brain. Subdural hemorrhage: Blood pools between the skull and the surface of the brain.

Isolette: A clear plastic enclosed crib that maintains a warm environment for a new baby and isolates them from germs.

Motor delay: A developmental delay that affects a person's muscle coordination. Includes fine and gross motor skills.

Nocturnal enuresis: Involuntary urination during sleep when a person is past the age of toilet training.

Obsessive Compulsive Disorder (OCD): Features a pattern of unwanted thoughts and fears known as obsessions. These obsessions lead to repetitive behaviors, also called compulsions. These obsessions and compulsions get in the way of daily activities and cause distress. (Mayo Clinic)

Occipital bone: Forms the back and base of the skull.

Occupational therapy: An intervention that uses everyday life activities (occupations) to promote health, well-being, and the ability to participate in important activities. (American Occupational Therapy Association)

Parietal skull: Part of the skull roof consisting of two parietal bones that come together along the sagittal suture and attach to the temporal bones on both sides of the skull.

Perinatal asphyxia: An inadequate intake of oxygen of the baby during the birthing process.

Physical therapy: Treatment provided by a physical therapist or physical therapist assistant that helps improve movement and physical function, manage pain and other chronic conditions, and recover from and prevent injury and chronic disease. (American Physical Therapy Association)

Pleural effusion: "Water on the lungs." A buildup of excess fluid between the layers of the pleura outside the lungs. (Cleveland Clinic)

Post-traumatic stress disorder (PTSD): A mental health condition triggered by a terrifying event — either experiencing it or witnessing it. Symptoms may include flashbacks, nightmares and severe anxiety, as well as uncontrollable thoughts about the event. (Mayo Clinic)

Respiratory syncytial virus (RSV): A viral illness that causes breathing problems. Can lead to severe respiratory illness and pneumonia in high-risk babies that can develop into asthma as they age.

Response to Intervention (RTI): A prevention model to limit or prevent academic failure for students who are having difficulty learning by providing "scientific research-based interventions" to bring students up to grade level achievement. (Learning Disabilities Association of America)

Retroperitoneal hematoma: A rare but potentially life-threatening condition that can occur after trauma. A collection of blood in the retroperitoneal space, which is behind the peritoneal cavity and in the back of the abdomen.

Sensory disorder and diet: A neurological condition that interferes with the body's ability to receive messages from the senses and convert those messages into appropriate motor and behavioral responses. A sensory diet is an individualized plan of physical activities and accommodations to help a person meet their sensory needs. (Autism Awareness Centre)

Speech-language pathologist (SLP): A licensed professional who is an expert in communication and treats those who have speech, language, voice, fluency, and swallowing disorders.

Speech delay: A developmental delay in a person's speech compared to those who are of similar age.

Subarachnoid hemorrhage (SAH): Bleeding into the subarachnoid space, which is the area between the brain and the tissues that cover it.

Subchorionic placental hemorrhage: When blood collects under the chorion membrane during pregnancy. This membrane attaches the mother's uterine wall to her baby's amniotic sac. (Cleveland Clinic)

Ventriculoperitoneal (VP) shunt: A surgically implanted device, with a thin plastic tube shaped much like a straw, that assists in draining CSF from the brain. Treats hydrocephalus.

www.ingramcontent.com/pod-product-compliance
Lightning Source LLC
Chambersburg PA
CBHW051611120626
46551CB00014B/1753